FITNESS AND EXERCISE
SOURCEBOOK

SEVENTH EDITION

Health Reference Series

FITNESS AND EXERCISE
SOURCEBOOK

SEVENTH EDITION

Basic Consumer Health Information on the Benefits of Physical Fitness, including Strength, Endurance, Longevity, Weight Management, Bone Health, and Stress Management, with Exercise Guidelines for All Ages, Tips on Maintaining Motivation, Measuring Exercise Intensity, Preventing Injuries, and Exercising with Health Conditions

Along with Information on Exercise Equipment, Fitness Tourism, Wearable Technology, a Glossary of Related Terms, and a Directory of Resources for Additional Help and Information

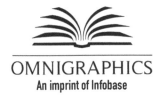

OMNIGRAPHICS
An imprint of Infobase

Bibliographic Note

Because this page cannot legibly accommodate all the copyright notices, the Bibliographic Note portion of the Preface constitutes an extension of the copyright notice.

* * *

OMNIGRAPHICS
An imprint of Infobase
8 The Green
Suite #19225
Dover, DE 19901
www.infobase.com
James Chambers, *Editorial Director*

* * *

Copyright © 2025 Infobase
ISBN 978-0-7808-2156-9
E-ISBN 978-0-7808-2157-6

Library of Congress Cataloging-in-Publication Data

Names: Chambers, James, editor.

Title: Fitness and exercise sourcebook / edited by James Chambers.

Description: Seventh edition. | Dover, DE: Omnigraphics, An imprint of Infobase, 2025. | Series: Health reference series | Includes index. | Summary: "Provides basic consumer health information on physical fitness, along with the various types of exercises, guidelines for starting and maintaining an exercise program, and strategies to prevent injuries. Includes an index, glossary of related terms, and other resources"-- Provided by publisher.

Identifiers: LCCN 2024037376 (print) | LCCN 2024037377 (ebook) | ISBN 9780780821569 (library binding) | ISBN 9780780821576 (ebook)

Subjects: LCSH: Physical fitness--Handbooks, manuals, etc. | Exercise--Handbooks, manuals, etc.

Classification: LCC GV436 .F53 2025 (print) | LCC GV436 (ebook) | DDC 613.7--dc23/eng/20240919

LC record available at https://lccn.loc.gov/2024037376

LC ebook record available at https://lccn.loc.gov/2024037377

Electronic or mechanical reproduction, including photography, recording, or any other information storage and retrieval system for the purpose of resale is strictly prohibited without permission in writing from the publisher.

The information in this publication was compiled from the sources cited and from other sources considered reliable. While every possible effort has been made to ensure reliability, the publisher will not assume liability for damages caused by inaccuracies in the data, and makes no warranty, express or implied, on the accuracy of the information contained herein.

This book is printed on acid-free paper meeting the ANSI Z39.48 Standard. The infinity symbol that appears above indicates that the paper in this book meets that standard.

Printed in the United States

Table of Contents

Preface..xi

Part 1. Introduction to Fitness
Chapter 1—Physical Activity: An Overview 3
Chapter 2—The Importance of Physical Activity 9
Chapter 3—The Four Essential Types of Exercise 13
Chapter 4—Physical Activity and Mental Health 17
  Section 4.1—Promoting Brain Health through
        Physical Activity 19
  Section 4.2—Role of Physical Activity in Mood
        Regulation...22
  Section 4.3—Exercise and Its Role in Preventing
        Cognitive Decline 26
  Section 4.4—Light Exercise: A Key to Boosting
        Memory and Brain Health 29
Chapter 5—The Role of Physical Activity in Health and
    Weight Management..33
Chapter 6—Myths about Nutrition and Physical Activity............39
Chapter 7—Physical Inactivity Trends among Adults
    50 Years and Older 43

Part 2. Guidelines for Lifelong Physical Fitness
Chapter 8—Understanding the Physical Activity Guidelines
    for Americans 51
Chapter 9—Physical Fitness for Children....................................55
  Section 9.1—Physical Activity Guidelines and
        Benefits for Children 57
  Section 9.2—Physical Activity for Preschoolers 60

v

    Section 9.3—Physical Education and Physical
         Activity in Schools 62
    Section 9.4—School Guidelines for Health
         and Fitness 65
Chapter 10—Physical Fitness for Teenagers 69
Chapter 11—Promoting Physical Activity in Youth 73
    Section 11.1—Physical Activity Guidelines for
         Children and Adolescents 75
    Section 11.2—The Role of Physical Activity in
         Youth Health and Academic Success 79
    Section 11.3—Benefits of Physical Activity
         for Girls 81
    Section 11.4—Balancing Screen Time and Physical
         Activity for a Healthy Lifestyle 83
Chapter 12—Physical Fitness for Adults 87
    Section 12.1—Key Guidelines for Physical
         Activity in Adults 89
    Section 12.2—Preventing Heart Disease in
         Women through Physical Activity 93
    Section 12.3—Physical Activity during Pregnancy
         and Postpartum 96
    Section 12.4—Physical Activity and the Menstrual
         Cycle 99
    Section 12.5—Managing Weight and Health
         through Physical Activity 101
Chapter 13—Physical Fitness for Older Adults 105
    Section 13.1—Promoting Physical Activity
         for Healthy Aging 107
    Section 13.2—Exercise and Well-Being for
         Older Adults 111
    Section 13.3—Ensuring Safety in Physical
         Activity for Older Adults 115
    Section 13.4—Safety Tips for Exercising
         Outdoors for Older Adults 119
    Section 13.5—The Heart Benefits of Light
         Physical Activity for Older Women 121

Part 3. Start Moving

Chapter 14—Building an Active Lifestyle 127
        Section 14.1—Incorporating Physical Activity into Daily Life 129
        Section 14.2—Getting Active and Overcoming Physical Activity Roadblocks 133
        Section 14.3—Making Exercise a Shared Enjoyment 136
Chapter 15—Staying Active and Eating Right 139
Chapter 16—Creating and Sticking to a Fitness Plan 143
        Section 16.1—Building Sustainable Exercise Habits 145
        Section 16.2—Goal Setting for Physical Activity Success 147
Chapter 17—Strategies for Prompts to Encourage Physical Activity 151
Chapter 18—Overcoming Obstacles to Physical Activity 155
Chapter 19—Measuring Health and Fitness 159
        Section 19.1—Heart Rate Targets for Fitness 161
        Section 19.2—Body Mass Index (BMI) for Health Assessment 164
        Section 19.3—Energy Balance and Weight Management 168
Chapter 20—Choosing Fitness Partners 171
        Section 20.1—Supporting Loved Ones in Staying Active 173
        Section 20.2—Family Fitness through Fun and Engaging Activities 175
Chapter 21—Roles and Responsibilities of Fitness Trainers and Instructors 179
Chapter 22—Debunking Weight Loss Myths and Scams 181

Part 4. Categories of Exercise or Physical Fitness

Chapter 23—Aerobic Activity 187
Chapter 24—Martial Arts for Youth 191

Chapter 25—Aquatic Exercise 195
        Section 25.1—Benefits and Safety of Water-
                Based Exercise 197
        Section 25.2—Swimming Risks and Safety
                Measures 198
Chapter 26—Walking and Hiking..201
        Section 26.1—Enhancing Physical Activity and
                Health through Walking 203
        Section 26.2—Hiking with Friends and Family........205
Chapter 27—Bicycling...209
        Section 27.1—Bicycling Basics....................................211
        Section 27.2—Bicycling Safety 212
Chapter 28—Strength and Resistance Training 217
        Section 28.1—Basics of Resistance Training 219
        Section 28.2—Strength Training for
                Healthier Aging..................................221
Chapter 29—Flexibility..225
Chapter 30—Mind-Body Exercises 229
        Section 30.1—Exploring Mind and Body
                Practices..231
        Section 30.2—Yoga for Health and Wellness 233
        Section 30.3—Tai Chi and Qigong 237
        Section 30.4—Meditation and Mindfulness..............241

Part 5. Fitness Safety
Chapter 31—Workout Safety 247
        Section 31.1—The Essentials of Warming
                Up and Cooling Down......................249
        Section 31.2—Common Workout Mistakes and
                How to Avoid Them 252
        Section 31.3—Physical Activity and Proper Gear 254
Chapter 32—Nutrition and Exercise 259
        Section 32.1—Hydration and Health 261
        Section 32.2—Nutrition for an Active Lifestyle........263
        Section 32.3—Dietary Supplements for Exercise......266

Section 32.4—Anabolic Steroids and Other
                Performance-Enhancing Drugs........269
Section 32.5—The Risks of Bodybuilding
                Products Containing Steroids...........274
Chapter 33—Guide to Sports Injury Management......................277
Section 33.1—Understanding and Managing
                Sports Injuries.....................................279
Section 33.2—Diagnosis, Treatment, and
                Management of Sports Injuries.........281
Section 33.3—Understanding and Managing
                Concussions in Teens.........................285
Chapter 34—Exercising Outdoors in Polluted Air.....................289

Part 6. Physical Fitness for Health Conditions
Chapter 35—Physical Activity for Chronic Conditions................293
Chapter 36—Fitness for People with Disabilities.......................297
Section 36.1—Healthy Living for People with
                Disabilities...299
Section 36.2—Staying Active with a Disability........301
Chapter 37—Fitness for Overweight Individuals 305
Section 37.1—Overweight, Obesity, and the
                Role of Physical Activity....................307
Section 37.2—Physical Activity for People of
                All Sizes..309
Chapter 38—Cardiac Rehabilitation for Heart Health
                Recovery..315
Chapter 39—Fitness for Bone Disorders...319
Section 39.1—Managing Arthritis with
                Physical Activity..................................321
Section 39.2—Preventing Osteoporosis through
                Exercise 324
Section 39.3—Managing Osteogenesis Imperfecta....327
Chapter 40—Fitness for Asthma...331
Chapter 41—Managing Diabetes through Physical Activity........335
Chapter 42—Physical Activity and Cancer.................................339

Chapter 43—Overcoming the Challenges of an Inactive
            Lifestyle 345
Chapter 44—The Benefits of Quitting Smoking for Fitness
            and Health..349
Chapter 45—The Importance of Quality Sleep for Well-Being........353

Part 7. Health and Wellness Trends
Chapter 46—Top Fitness Trends of 2023 361
Chapter 47—Wellness Tourism..363
Chapter 48—Smart Devices for Better Health Monitoring...........367
Chapter 49—Improving Wellness Care through Technology 371

Part 8. Additional Help and Information
Chapter 50—Glossary of Terms Related to Fitness and Exercise......377
Chapter 51—Directory of Fitness Resources....................................383

Index 393

Preface

ABOUT THIS BOOK
Regular physical activity provides numerous health benefits, including reducing the risk of chronic conditions such as diabetes, heart disease, obesity, osteoporosis, and certain cancers. It also promotes mental well-being, longevity, and overall life satisfaction. Despite these benefits, only 24.2 percent of U.S. adults aged 18 and over met the *Physical Activity Guidelines for Americans* for both aerobic and muscle-strengthening activities in 2020. This gap highlights the ongoing challenges in promoting regular exercise, even though it could prevent approximately 1 in 10 premature deaths.

Fitness and Exercise Sourcebook, Seventh Edition offers a comprehensive guide to the health benefits of physical activity, with tailored recommendations for people of all ages, including those with disabilities and chronic health conditions. The book offers practical tips for incorporating fitness into daily routines, setting achievable goals, and staying motivated. It covers a variety of physical activities, including aerobic, strength, balance, and mind-body exercises, while also addressing important safety considerations and providing guidance on nutrition, hydration, and equipment. The book concludes with a glossary of related terms and a directory of resources for further assistance and information.

HOW TO USE THIS BOOK
This book is divided into parts and chapters. Parts focus on broad areas of interest. Chapters are devoted to single topics within a part.

Part 1: Introduction to Fitness explains the physical and mental benefits of regular physical activity, focusing on its role in preventing diseases, enhancing mental well-being, improving memory, and maintaining a healthy weight. This part provides an overview of different types of exercises and highlights the importance of incorporating daily exercise to maximize longevity.

Part 2: Guidelines for Lifelong Physical Fitness offers fitness recommendations tailored for various age groups, including children, teenagers, adults, and older adults. It includes practical tips for promoting lifelong physical activity and emphasizes the significance of staying active to prevent inactivity-related health issues, especially among adults over 50.

Part 3: Start Moving provides guidance on integrating physical activity into everyday life, creating and adhering to a fitness plan, and overcoming common barriers to exercise. It includes tips on selecting fitness partners, tracking exercise intensity, and choosing suitable fitness equipment.

Part 4: Categories of Exercise or Physical Fitness explores various exercise forms, including aerobic activities, strength training, walking, biking, and mind-body practices such as yoga, tai chi, and Pilates. This part explains how each type contributes to overall fitness and well-being, offering insights into their specific benefits.

Part 5: Fitness Safety focuses on safe exercise practices, offering tips on avoiding common workout mistakes, choosing proper equipment, staying hydrated, and maintaining proper nutrition. It addresses injury prevention, the dangers of overtraining, and precautions for exercising outdoors, particularly in extreme weather.

Part 6: Physical Fitness for Health Conditions provides exercise recommendations for individuals with specific health conditions, including disabilities, obesity, heart disease, bone disorders, respiratory issues, diabetes, and cancer. It emphasizes the role of physical activity in managing these conditions and improving overall health.

Part 7: Health and Wellness Trends examines current trends in the fitness and wellness industry, including the top fitness trends of 2023. It discusses the growing interest in wellness tourism, the use of smart devices for health monitoring, and how technology is improving wellness care.

Part 8: Additional Help and Information includes a glossary of important fitness-related terms and a directory of organizations offering information and resources on physical fitness and exercise.

BIBLIOGRAPHIC NOTE

This volume contains documents and excerpts from publications issued by the following U.S. government agencies: Centers for Disease Control and Prevention (CDC); Federal Trade Commission (FTC); girlshealth.gov;

MedlinePlus; National Cancer Institute (NCI); National Center for Complementary and Integrative Health (NCCIH); National Heart, Lung, and Blood Institute (NHLBI); National Highway Traffic Safety Administration (NHTSA); National Institute of Arthritis and Musculoskeletal and Skin Diseases (NIAMS); National Institute of Biomedical Imaging and Bioengineering (NIBIB); National Institute of Diabetes and Digestive and Kidney Diseases (NIDDK); National Institute on Aging (NIA); National Institutes of Health (NIH); Office of Disease Prevention and Health Promotion (ODPHP); Office on Women's Health (OWH); Smokefree.gov; U.S. Bureau of Labor Statistics (BLS); U.S. Department of Veterans Affairs (VA); U.S. Environmental Protection Agency (EPA); U.S. Food and Drug Administration (FDA); U.S. Forest Service (USFS); and U.S. Government Publishing Office (GPO).

ABOUT THE *HEALTH REFERENCE SERIES*

The *Health Reference Series* is designed to provide basic medical information for patients, families, caregivers, and the general public. Each volume provides comprehensive coverage on a particular topic. This is especially important for people who may be dealing with a newly diagnosed disease or a chronic disorder in themselves or in a family member. People looking for preventive guidance, information about disease warning signs, medical statistics, and risk factors for health problems will also find answers to their questions in the *Health Reference Series*. The *Series*, however, is not intended to serve as a tool for diagnosing illness, in prescribing treatments, or as a substitute for the physician-patient relationship. All people concerned about medical symptoms or the possibility of disease are encouraged to seek professional care from an appropriate health-care provider.

A NOTE ABOUT SPELLING AND STYLE

Health Reference Series editors use *Stedman's Medical Dictionary* as an authority for questions related to the spelling of medical terms and *The Chicago Manual of Style* for questions related to grammatical structures, punctuation, and other editorial concerns. Consistent adherence is not always possible, however, because the individual volumes within the *Series* include many documents from a wide variety of different producers, and the editor's primary goal is to present material from each source as accurately as is possible. This sometimes means that information in different chapters or sections may follow other guidelines and alternate spelling authorities. For example, occasionally a copyright holder may require that eponymous terms be shown in possessive forms (Crohn's disease vs. Crohn disease) or that British spelling norms be retained (leukaemia vs. leukemia).

HEALTH REFERENCE SERIES UPDATE POLICY

The inaugural book in the *Health Reference Series* was the first edition of *Cancer Sourcebook* published in 1989. Since then, the *Series* has been enthusiastically received by librarians and in the medical community. In order to maintain the standard of providing high-quality health information for the layperson, the editorial staff felt it was necessary to implement a policy of updating volumes when warranted.

Medical researchers have been making tremendous strides, and it is the purpose of the *Health Reference Series* to stay current with the most recent advances. Each decision to update a volume is made on an individual basis. Some of the considerations include how much new information is available and the feedback we receive from people who use the books. If there is a topic you would like to see added to the update list, or an area of medical concern you feel has not been adequately addressed, please write to: custserv@infobaselearning.com.

Part 1 | Introduction to Fitness

Chapter 1 | Physical Activity: An Overview

WHAT IS PHYSICAL ACTIVITY?
Physical activity is any body movement that works your muscles and requires more energy than resting. Walking, running, dancing, swimming, yoga, and gardening are a few examples of physical activity. According to the *Physical Activity Guidelines for Americans*, physical activity generally refers to movement that enhances health. It is recommended for everyone aged three and older.

TYPES OF PHYSICAL ACTIVITY
The three main types of physical activity are aerobic, muscle-strengthening, and bone-strengthening. Balance and flexibility activities are also beneficial. Aerobic activity benefits your heart and lungs the most. By understanding the different types of physical activity, their benefits, and recommendations, you can create a plan to add physical activity to your healthy lifestyle.

Aerobic Activity
Aerobic activity moves your large muscles, such as those in your arms and legs. Aerobic activity is also called "endurance activity."

Aerobic activity makes your heart beat faster than usual. You also breathe harder during this type of activity. Over time, regular aerobic activity makes your heart and lungs stronger and able to work better.

Fitness and Exercise Sourcebook, Seventh Edition

Muscle-Strengthening Activity
Muscle-strengthening activities improve muscle strength, power, and endurance. Push-ups and sit-ups, lifting weights, climbing stairs, and digging in the garden are examples of muscle-strengthening activities.

Bone-Strengthening Activity
With bone-strengthening activities, your feet, legs, or arms support your body's weight, and your muscles push against your bones. This helps make your bones strong. Running, walking, jumping rope, and lifting weights are examples of bone-strengthening activities.

Muscle-strengthening and bone-strengthening activities can also be aerobic, depending on whether they make your heart and lungs work harder than usual. For example, running is both an aerobic activity and a bone-strengthening activity.

Balance Activities
These kinds of activities can improve your ability to resist forces that can make you fall, either while stationary or moving. Walking backward, standing on one leg, walking heel-to-toe, practicing standing from a sitting position, or using a wobble board are examples of balance activities. Strengthening the muscles of the back, abdomen, and legs also improves balance.

Flexibility Activities
Stretching helps improve your flexibility and your ability to fully move your joints. Touching your toes, doing side stretches, and doing yoga exercises are examples of stretching.[1]

PHYSICAL EXERCISE
How Does Regular Exercise Benefit You?
When you hear the word "exercise," you might think about lifting weights or using a treadmill to try to lose a few pounds. Weight loss

---

[1] "What Is Physical Activity?" National Heart, Lung, and Blood Institute (NHLBI), March 24, 2022. Available online. URL: www.nhlbi.nih.gov/health/heart/physical-activity. Accessed September 4, 2024.

Physical Activity: An Overview

can be one benefit of getting enough physical activity, but there are other important ways that exercise helps you stay healthy, including physical, emotional, and mental benefits.

Regular exercise can help you stay physically healthy by:
- **Building strength.** Stronger muscles help with performing everyday activities.
- **Helping to manage and even prevent some diseases.** Exercise can help manage and prevent conditions such as arthritis, heart disease, stroke, and type 2 diabetes.
- **Helping you lose weight or keep you from gaining weight.** Regular exercise contributes to maintaining a healthy weight.
- **Giving you more energy and making you feel less tired.** Staying active can improve energy levels.
- **Enabling you to sleep better.** Physical activity can promote better sleep.
- **Helping with balance and preventing falls.** Exercise improves balance and coordination, reducing the risk of falls.

Emotional and mental benefits of exercise include:
- **Less stress, anxiety, and depression.** Exercise can help manage stress and improve mood.
- **Feeling more in control.** Regular physical activity can enhance a sense of control over one's life.
- **Improved self-esteem.** Engaging in physical activity can boost self-confidence.
- **Finding it easier to plan, focus, and shift between tasks.** Exercise can improve cognitive function.
- **Enhanced reasoning and thinking.** Regular activity may improve overall mental sharpness.
- **Possibly lowered risk of developing Alzheimer disease (AD).** Some research suggests that exercise may reduce the risk of cognitive decline.

Being Active: How Much Is Enough?

Guidance from your health-care provider can help determine how much activity is right for you based on your lifestyle. Here are some general suggestions:

- **60 minutes.** The amount of daily moderate to vigorous activity children and teens should get. This includes activities such as walking, running, and sports that make the heart beat faster. Adults who want to lose or maintain weight should aim for this amount as well.
- **150 minutes.** The minimum amount of weekly moderate activity adults should get to stay healthy. Strengthening activities should also be included two or more days a week.
- **Moderate activity.** Activities include walking, biking, jogging, volleyball, climbing stairs, gardening, raking leaves, and dancing. A good test is to try to talk while doing the activity. Making conversation might be a little more difficult, but you should not be gasping for air.
- **Vigorous activity.** Activities include hiking, running, shoveling snow, carrying heavy loads, basketball, soccer, bicycling, and singles tennis. Making conversation should be difficult at this level.
- **Strength exercises.** Activities include lifting weights using large muscles such as those in the arms or thighs, using resistance bands, and using your body weight by doing push-ups, pull-ups, crunches, and squats. These exercises strengthen large muscles or make your muscles work harder than usual. Doing these activities at least two days a week can help build strength and keep or increase muscle mass.[2]

Being physically active is one of the best ways to keep your heart and lungs healthy. Many Americans are not active enough.

---

[2] MedlinePlus, "Physical Exercise," National Institutes of Health (NIH), March 31, 2022. Available online. URL: https://magazine.medlineplus.gov/article/physical-exercise. Accessed September 4, 2024.

Physical Activity: An Overview

The good news, though, is that even modest amounts of physical activity are good for your health. The more active you are, the more you will benefit.[3]

---

[3] See footnote [1].

Chapter 2 | The Importance of Physical Activity

WHY IS PHYSICAL ACTIVITY IMPORTANT?
Exercise and physical activity are beneficial for almost everyone, including older adults. Regardless of your health and physical abilities, staying active can offer numerous advantages. In fact, studies show that "taking it easy" can be risky. Often, inactivity is more to blame than age when older people lose the ability to perform daily tasks independently. Lack of physical activity can also lead to more visits to the doctor, increased hospitalizations, and greater use of medications for various illnesses.

Including all four types of exercise (endurance, strength, balance, and flexibility) can benefit many areas of your life. Staying active can help you:
- keep and improve your strength
- have more energy
- boost your immune system
- improve your balance
- manage and prevent conditions such as arthritis, heart disease, stroke, type 2 diabetes, osteoporosis, and certain types of cancer, including breast and colon cancer
- sleep better
- reduce levels of stress and anxiety
- enhance your cognitive function
- reach or maintain a healthy weight
- control your blood pressure
- perk up your mood

Fitness and Exercise Sourcebook, Seventh Edition

EMOTIONAL BENEFITS OF EXERCISE

Research shows that exercise not only benefits physical health but also supports emotional and mental health. Exercising with a friend can provide the added benefit of emotional support. The next time you feel down, anxious, or stressed, try to get up and start moving!

Physical activity can help:
- reduce feelings of depression and stress
- increase your energy level
- improve sleep
- empower you to feel more in control

Additionally, exercise and physical activity may improve or maintain some aspects of cognitive function, such as the ability to switch quickly between tasks, plan activities, and ignore irrelevant information.

Here are some exercise ideas to help lift your mood:
- **Walking, bicycling, or dancing**. Endurance activities increase your breathing, get your heart pumping, and boost chemicals in your body that may improve mood.
- **Yoga**. This mind-body practice typically combines physical postures, breathing exercises, and relaxation.
- **Tai chi**. This "moving meditation" involves shifting the body slowly, gently, and precisely while breathing deeply.
- **Activities you enjoy**. Whether it is gardening, playing tennis, or kicking a soccer ball with your grandchildren, choose activities you want to do, not activities you feel you have to do.[1]

THE HEALTH BENEFITS OF PHYSICAL ACTIVITY

Research demonstrates that participating in regular moderate-to-vigorous physical activity provides many health benefits. Some benefits of physical activity can be achieved immediately, such as reduced feelings of anxiety, reduced blood pressure, and improvements in sleep, cognitive function, and insulin sensitivity. Other

---

[1] National Institute on Aging (NIA), "Real-Life Benefits of Exercise and Physical Activity," National Institutes of Health (NIH), April 3, 2020. Available online. URL: www.nia.nih.gov/health/exercise-and-physical-activity/real-life-benefits-exercise-and-physical-activity. Accessed September 4, 2024.

The Importance of Physical Activity

benefits, such as increased cardiorespiratory fitness, increased muscular strength, decreased depressive symptoms, and sustained reduction in blood pressure, require a few weeks or months of participation in physical activity. Physical activity can also slow or delay the progression of chronic diseases such as hypertension and type 2 diabetes. These benefits persist with continued physical activity.

The health benefits of physical activity are observed in children and adolescents, young and middle-aged adults, older adults, women and men, people of different races and ethnicities, and people with chronic conditions or disabilities. The health benefits of physical activity are generally independent of body weight. Adults of all sizes and shapes gain health and fitness benefits by being habitually physically active. The benefits of physical activity also outweigh the risks of injury and heart attacks, two concerns that may prevent people from becoming physically active.

Children and Adolescents
- improved bone health (ages 3–17 years)
- improved weight status (ages 3–17 years)
- improved cardiorespiratory and muscular fitness (ages 6–17 years)
- improved cardiometabolic health (ages 6–17 years)
- reduced risk of depression (ages 6–13 years)

Adults and Older Adults
- lower risk of all-cause mortality
- lower risk of cardiovascular disease mortality
- lower risk of cardiovascular disease (including heart disease and stroke)
- lower risk of hypertension
- lower risk of type 2 diabetes
- lower risk of adverse blood lipid profile
- lower risk of cancers of the bladder, breast, colon, endometrium, esophagus, kidney, lung, and stomach
- reduced risk of dementia (including Alzheimer disease (AD))
- improved quality of life (QOL)

Fitness and Exercise Sourcebook, Seventh Edition

- reduced anxiety
- reduced risk of depression
- improved sleep
- slowed or reduced weight gain
- weight loss, particularly when combined with reduced calorie intake
- prevention of weight regain following initial weight loss
- improved bone health
- improved physical function
- lower risk of falls (older adults)
- lower risk of fall-related injuries (older adults)

MAJOR RESEARCH FINDINGS

- Regular moderate-to-vigorous physical activity reduces the risk of many adverse health outcomes.
- Some physical activity is better than none.
- For most health outcomes, additional benefits occur as the amount of physical activity increases through higher intensity, greater frequency, and/or longer duration.
- Substantial health benefits for adults occur with 150–300 minutes a week of moderate-intensity physical activity, such as brisk walking. Additional benefits occur with more physical activity.
- Both aerobic and muscle-strengthening physical activities are beneficial.
- Health benefits occur for children and adolescents, young and middle-aged adults, older adults, and those in every studied racial and ethnic group.
- The health benefits of physical activity occur for people with chronic conditions or disabilities.
- The benefits of physical activity generally outweigh the risks of adverse outcomes or injury.[2]

---

[2] Office of Disease Prevention and Health Promotion (ODPHP), "Current Guidelines," U.S. Department of Health and Human Services (HHS), August 24, 2021. Available online. URL: https://health.gov/our-work/nutrition-physical-activity/physical-activity-guidelines/current-guidelines. Accessed September 4, 2024.

Chapter 3 | The Four Essential Types of Exercise

THE IMPORTANCE OF A WELL-ROUNDED EXERCISE ROUTINE
Most people tend to focus on one type of exercise or activity and think they are doing enough. However, research has shown that it is important to incorporate all four types of exercise: endurance, strength, balance, and flexibility. Each type offers different benefits. Engaging in one kind of exercise can also improve your ability to perform others, and variety helps reduce boredom and the risk of injury. Regardless of your age, you can find activities that meet your fitness level and needs.

ENDURANCE EXERCISE
Endurance activities, often referred to as "aerobic exercises," increase your breathing and heart rates. These activities help keep you healthy, improve your fitness, and enable you to perform everyday tasks. Endurance exercises improve the health of your heart, lungs, and circulatory system. They can also delay or prevent many diseases common in older adults, such as diabetes, colon and breast cancers, heart disease, and others. Physical activities that build endurance include:
- brisk walking or jogging
- yard work (mowing, raking)
- dancing
- swimming

- biking
- climbing stairs or hills
- playing tennis or basketball

Aim for at least 150 minutes of activity each week that makes you breathe hard. To reach this goal, try to be active throughout your day and avoid sitting for long periods.

Safety Tips
- To warm up and cool down, do a little light activity, such as easy walking, before and after your endurance activities.
- Listen to your body: endurance activities should not cause dizziness, chest pain or pressure, or a sensation similar to heartburn.
- Be sure to drink liquids when doing any activity that makes you sweat. If your doctor has advised you to limit your fluid intake, check before increasing the amount of fluid you drink while exercising.
- If you are exercising outdoors, be aware of your surroundings.
- Dress in layers, so you can add or remove clothes as needed for hot and cold weather.
- To prevent injuries, use safety equipment, such as a helmet when bicycling.

STRENGTH EXERCISE
Your muscular strength can make a big difference in your daily life. Some people refer to using weights to improve muscle strength as "strength training" or "resistance training."

Some people choose to use weights to help improve their strength. If you do, start with light weights and gradually increase them. Other people use resistance bands, which are stretchy elastic bands available in varying strengths. If you are a beginner, try exercising without the band or use a light band until you are comfortable. Move on to a stronger band (or more weight) when you can do two sets of 10–15 repetitions easily. Try to do strength exercises for all major muscle groups at least two days per week, but avoid

The Four Essential Types of Exercise

exercising the same muscle group on consecutive days. Below are a few examples of strength exercises:
- lifting weights
- carrying groceries
- gripping a tennis ball
- overhead arm curl
- arm curls
- wall push-ups
- lifting your body weight
- using a resistance band

Safety Tips
- Do not hold your breath during strength exercises; breathe regularly.
- Breathe out as you lift or push, and breathe in as you relax.
- Talk with your doctor if you are unsure about doing a particular exercise.

BALANCE EXERCISES
Balance exercises help prevent falls, a common issue among older adults that can have serious consequences. Many lower-body strength exercises will also improve your balance. Balance exercises include:
- tai chi, a "moving meditation" that involves shifting the body slowly, gently, and precisely while breathing deeply
- standing on one foot
- the heel-to-toe walk
- the balance walk
- standing from a seated position

Safety Tips
- Have a sturdy chair or a person nearby to hold on to if you feel unsteady.
- Talk with your doctor if you are unsure about a particular exercise.

Fitness and Exercise Sourcebook, Seventh Edition

FLEXIBILITY EXERCISES

Stretching can improve your flexibility. Being more flexible will make it easier to reach down to tie your shoes or look over your shoulder when backing your car out of the driveway. Flexibility exercises include:
- the backstretch exercise
- the inner thigh stretch
- the ankle stretch
- the back of the leg stretch

Safety Tips
- Stretch when your muscles are warmed up.
- Stretch after endurance or strength exercises.
- Do not stretch so far that it hurts.
- Always remember to breathe normally while holding a stretch.
- Talk with your doctor if you are unsure about a particular exercise.[1]

---

[1] National Institute on Aging (NIA), "Four Types of Exercise Can Improve Your Health and Physical Ability," National Institutes of Health (NIH), January 29, 2021. Available online. URL: www.nia.nih.gov/health/exercise-and-physical-activity/four-types-exercise-can-improve-your-health-and-physical. Accessed September 3, 2024.

Chapter 4 | Physical Activity and Mental Health

Chapter Contents

Section 4.1—Promoting Brain Health through
 Physical Activity 19
Section 4.2—Role of Physical Activity in Mood Regulation 22
Section 4.3—Exercise and Its Role in Preventing
 Cognitive Decline 26
Section 4.4—Light Exercise: A Key to Boosting Memory
 and Brain Health 29

Section 4.1 | Promoting Brain Health through Physical Activity

DEFINING BRAIN HEALTH
Brain health can be defined in various ways, but the *Physical Activity Guidelines* focuses on the following areas:
- **Youth**. Brain maturation, development, and academic achievement.
- **Older adults**. Dementia and cognitive impairment.
- **Across the lifespan**. Cognition, anxiety and depression, quality of life (QOL), and sleep.

Some benefits of physical activity on brain health occur immediately after a session of moderate-to-vigorous physical activity (acute effect), such as reduced feelings of state anxiety (short-term anxiety), improved sleep, and enhanced aspects of cognitive function. With regular physical activity (habitual effect), improvements are observed in trait anxiety (long-term anxiety), deep sleep, and components of executive function, including the ability to plan and organize, monitor, inhibit or facilitate behaviors, initiate tasks, and control emotions.

Table 4.1 outlines the various benefits of physical activity on brain health, detailing the positive outcomes observed across different age groups and conditions, such as cognition, QOL, mood, anxiety, and sleep.[1]

Table 4.1. The Benefits of Physical Activity for Brain Health

Outcome	Population	Benefit
	Children aged 6–13 years	Improved cognition
	Adults	Reduced risk of dementia or Alzheimer disease (AD)
Cognition	Adults older than 50 years	Improved cognition

---

[1] Office of Disease Prevention and Health Promotion (ODPHP), "Current Guidelines," U.S. Department of Health and Human Services (HHS), August 24, 2021. Available online. URL: https://health.gov/our-work/nutrition-physical-activity/physical-activity-guidelines/current-guidelines. Accessed September 4, 2024.

Table 4.1. Continued

Outcome	Population	Benefit
Quality of life	Adults	Improved QOL
Depressed mood and depression	Children aged 6–17 years and adults	Reduced risk of depression Reduced depressed mood
Anxiety	Adults	Reduced short-term feelings of anxiety
	Adults	Reduced long-term feelings and signs of anxiety (trait anxiety) for people with and without anxiety disorders
	Adults	Improved sleep outcomes
Sleep	Adults	Improved sleep outcomes that increase with the duration of acute episode

COGNITIVE HEALTH AND OLDER ADULTS

Cognitive health is the ability to think, learn, and remember clearly, which is essential for effectively carrying out many everyday activities. Cognitive health is one aspect of overall brain health.

Various factors can influence cognitive health. Genetic, environmental, and lifestyle factors may contribute to a decline in thinking skills and the ability to perform daily tasks, such as driving, paying bills, taking medicine, and cooking. While genetic factors cannot be controlled, many environmental and lifestyle factors can be changed or managed.

Scientific research suggests that there are steps you can take to reduce your risk of cognitive decline and help maintain your cognitive health. Implementing these changes into your daily routine can support brain function now and in the future.

Take Care of Your Physical Health

Taking care of your physical health can also benefit your cognitive health. Consider the following steps:

- **Get recommended health screenings**. Regular check-ups can help identify issues early.
- **Manage chronic health problems**. Conditions such as high blood pressure (HBP), diabetes, depression, and high cholesterol can affect cognitive health.

Physical Activity and Mental Health

- **Consult your health-care provider about medications.** Discuss possible side effects on memory, sleep, and brain function.
- **Treat age-related sensory conditions.** Address hearing or vision loss to improve overall well-being.
- **Reduce the risk of falls and other accidents that could lead to brain injuries.**
- **Limit alcohol consumption.** Be aware that some medications can be dangerous when mixed with alcohol.
- **Quit smoking.** Avoid other nicotine products, such as chewing tobacco.
- **Follow a healthy diet.** Choose foods that are nutritionally dense, low in animal fats, and high in vitamins and fiber.
- **Get enough sleep.** Strive for a full seven to nine hours each night.

Be Physically Active

Engaging in physical activity—whether through regular exercise, household chores, or other activities—provides numerous benefits. Physical activities can help you:
- maintain and improve your strength
- have more energy
- improve your balance
- prevent or delay heart disease, diabetes, and other health issues
- improve your mood and reduce depression

Several studies have supported a connection between physical activity and brain health. For example:
- One study found that higher levels of a protein that boosts brain health were present in both mice and humans who were more physically active than their sedentary peers.
- An observational study with cognitively normal, late-middle-aged participants found that more time spent engaging in moderate levels of physical activity was

associated with a greater increase in brain glucose metabolism—how quickly the brain turns glucose into fuel—which may reduce the risk of developing AD.
- A randomized controlled trial showed that exercise could increase the size of a brain structure important for memory and learning, leading to better spatial memory.

Although these results are encouraging, more research is needed to determine the specific role that exercise may play in preventing cognitive decline.

FEDERAL RECOMMENDATIONS FOR PHYSICAL ACTIVITY

Federal guidelines recommend that all adults engage in at least 150 minutes (2.5 hours) of physical activity each week. Walking is a good starting point. Additionally, joining programs that teach how to move safely and prevent falls can be beneficial, as falls can lead to serious injuries, including brain injuries. If you are not currently active but want to start a vigorous exercise program, consult your health-care provider.[2]

Section 4.2 | Role of Physical Activity in Mood Regulation

Physical activity can significantly improve your health and quality of life (QOL). Not getting enough physical activity increases your risk for conditions such as diabetes, heart disease, cancer, and mental health disorders.

STUDY OVERVIEW AND FINDINGS

A team led by Dr. Kathleen Merikangas at National Institutes of Health's (NIH) National Institute of Mental Health (NIMH) and

---

[2] National Institute on Aging (NIA), "Cognitive Health and Older Adults," National Institutes of Health (NIH), June 11, 2024. Available online. URL: www.nia.nih.gov/health/brain-health/cognitive-health-and-older-adults. Accessed September 4, 2024.

Physical Activity and Mental Health

Dr. Vadim Zipunnikov at Johns Hopkins University explored the relationship between mood disorders, physical activity, and sleep. They enrolled 54 adults with bipolar disorder, 91 with major depressive disorder, and 97 with no history of mood disorders. The study, supported in part by NIMH, was published online on December 12, 2018, in *JAMA Psychiatry*.

Over two weeks, participants wore mobile devices around their wrists to monitor physical activity and estimate sleep duration. They also kept a diary of their mood and energy levels four times a day, rating how they felt from "very happy" to "very sad" and "very tired" to "very energetic."

The researchers found that physical activity positively affected participants' mood, but mood did not influence the amount of physical activity they engaged in later. Physical activity also affected how energetic participants felt and the duration of their sleep. These relationships were reciprocal: energy levels and sleep also influenced how much physical activity participants engaged in afterward. The relationships among physical activity, sleep, mood, and energy were significantly stronger in people with bipolar-I disorder.[1]

MENTAL HEALTH BENEFITS OF PHYSICAL ACTIVITY

Physical activity offers many well-established mental health benefits, as noted in the *Physical Activity Guidelines for Americans*. These benefits include improved brain health and cognitive function, reduced risk of anxiety and depression, improved sleep, and overall enhanced QOL. Although not a cure-all, increasing physical activity directly contributes to improved mental health and overall health and well-being.

BOOSTING MENTAL AND PHYSICAL HEALTH THROUGH ACTIVITY

Everyone has their own way to "recharge" their sense of well-being—something that makes them feel good physically, emotionally, and

---

[1] News and Events, "Physical Activity May Reduce Depression Symptoms," National Institutes of Health (NIH), January 15, 2019. Available online. URL: www.nih.gov/news-events/nih-research-matters/physical-activity-helps-reduce-depression-symptoms. Accessed September 4, 2024.

spiritually, even if they are not consciously aware of it. For some, a walk around the block, a few push-ups, or a hike through the woods can quickly improve their day.

Knowing what physical activities make you feel better can change your day and life. Physical health is closely connected to mental health, and engaging in activities that improve physical health can also enhance mental well-being.

THE IMPORTANCE OF REGULAR PHYSICAL ACTIVITY

Approximately half of all people in the United States will be diagnosed with a mental health disorder at some point in their lifetime, with anxiety and anxiety disorders being the most common. Major depression is another common mental health disorder and a leading cause of disability for middle-aged adults. Compounding these issues, mental health disorders can affect a person's ability to engage in health-promoting behaviors, including physical activity.

The coronavirus 2019 (COVID-19) pandemic has underscored the need to prioritize physical and emotional health. The U.S. Surgeon General recently highlighted how the pandemic has exacerbated the mental health crisis among youth, highlighting the increased need for mental health awareness and care.

The good news is that even small amounts of physical activity can immediately reduce symptoms of anxiety in adults and older adults. Research suggests that increasing physical activity, regardless of type, can improve depression symptoms across the lifespan. Regular physical activity has also been shown to reduce the risk of developing depression in both children and adults.

ADAPTING PHYSICAL ACTIVITY TO CHANGING SEASONS

While the seasons and life circumstances may change, our basic needs remain the same. Just as we adapt our clothing and diet to the changing seasons, we must also adjust our approach to staying physically active. Sometimes this means bundling up for a walk in cold weather, wearing appropriate shoes, or finding creative ways to stay active indoors.

If weather or other conditions prevent a trip to the gym or a walk outside, consider other options such as impromptu dance parties at home or engaging in household chores. During the COVID-19 pandemic, many people built makeshift home gyms to stay active, saving time and money while maintaining muscle strength.

RECOMMENDATIONS FOR PHYSICAL ACTIVITY

The *Physical Activity Guidelines for Americans* recommends that adults engage in at least 150 minutes of moderate-intensity aerobic activity (anything that gets your heart beating faster) each week and include muscle-strengthening activities on at least two days per week. Youth need 60 minutes or more of physical activity each day. Preschool-aged children (ages three to five years) should be active throughout the day, with adult caregivers encouraging active play to support growth and development. Striving toward these goals and consistently engaging in physical activity can lead to better health outcomes both immediately and over the long term.

PHYSICAL ACTIVITY AND YOUTH MENTAL HEALTH

For youth, sports provide additional opportunities for physical activity and improved mental health. Participation in sports can offer psychological health benefits beyond those gained from other forms of leisure-time physical activity. These benefits include higher levels of perceived competence, confidence, and self-esteem, along with team-building, leadership, and resilience skills. Research has also shown that participation in youth sports is associated with a reduced risk of suicide and suicidal thoughts. Moreover, involvement in team sports during adolescence may lead to better mental health outcomes in adulthood, particularly for those who have experienced adverse childhood experiences. Besides the physical and mental health benefits, sports can simply be enjoyable.

BROADER IMPLICATIONS OF PHYSICAL ACTIVITY

The implications of physical activity for mental health and social well-being are vast, affecting every aspect of life. Recognizing this, the President's Council on Sports, Fitness, and Nutrition explicitly aims to expand national awareness of the importance of mental health as it relates to physical fitness and nutrition. While physical activity is not a substitute for mental health treatment when needed, it plays a vital role in supporting emotional and cognitive well-being.[2]

Section 4.3 | Exercise and Its Role in Preventing Cognitive Decline

THE ROLE OF PHYSICAL ACTIVITY IN PREVENTING HIPPOCAMPAL ATROPHY

Physical activity may help prevent atrophy of the hippocampus, a brain region critical for learning and memory that often shrinks in the brains of people with Alzheimer disease (AD). A recent study that examined the rate of hippocampal atrophy over 18 months in cognitively normal older adults suggests that physical activity may help prevent or delay this AD-related change.

The National Institute on Aging (NIA)-funded study, conducted by researchers at the Cleveland Clinic's Schey Center for Cognitive Neuroimaging, is the first to demonstrate the protective effects of physical activity on the hippocampus in older adults at genetic risk for AD. This research adds to previous findings indicating that physical activity—ranging from gardening to walking to structured exercise programs—may benefit cognitive function in older adults.

STUDY DETAILS AND FINDINGS

Researchers studied 97 cognitively normal adults, aged 65–89, some of whom had a family history of dementia. Participants were divided into four groups based on their self-reported levels of physical activity (low or high) and the presence or absence of the apolipoprotein E (APOE) ε4 gene, the strongest known genetic risk factor for AD. Individuals with low physical activity reported walking or engaging in other low-intensity activities on two or fewer days per week. Those with

---

[2] Office of Disease Prevention and Health Promotion (ODPHP), "Physical Activity Is Good for the Mind and the Body," U.S. Department of Health and Human Services (HHS), December 15, 2021. Available online. URL: https://health.gov/news/202112/physical-activity-good-mind-and-body. Accessed September 4, 2024.

high activity reported participating in moderate or vigorous activities, such as brisk walking or swimming, on three or more days per week.

All participants underwent magnetic resonance imaging (MRI) to measure the size of the hippocampus—a part of the brain that shrinks as AD progresses—and other brain structures. Neurobehavioral testing was also conducted to assess cognition and daily functioning. MRI scans were performed at the start of the study and again after 18 months. At the end of the study, researchers found that the hippocampus size decreased by 3 percent in the group with high genetic risk and low physical activity. In contrast, hippocampal size remained stable in the group with low genetic risk and in participants with high genetic risk who were highly physically active. Physical activity did not appear to affect other brain areas, including the amygdala, thalamus, and cortical white matter.

While these findings are promising, more research is needed to confirm them. Researchers are eager to understand how physical activity influences hippocampal atrophy in individuals at high genetic risk for AD. Animal studies suggest several possibilities, including the effect of physical activity on cholinergic function, brain inflammation, and cerebral blood flow.[1]

STAYING PHYSICALLY ACTIVE: ALZHEIMER DISEASE AND RELATED DEMENTIAS

Researchers are exploring the benefits of exercise to delay mild cognitive impairment (MCI) in older adults and improve brain function in those who may be at risk for developing AD. Older adults with MCI may be able to safely engage in more vigorous forms of exercise, similar to older adults without MCI, as long as there are no other underlying health concerns.

Being active and exercising can help people with AD or another form of dementia feel better. It can also help them maintain a healthy weight and regular toilet and sleep habits. For caregivers, exercising together can make physical activity more enjoyable.

---

[1] National Institute on Aging (NIA), "Physical Activity and Alzheimer-Related Hippocampal Atrophy," National Institutes of Health (NIH), August 4, 2014. Available online. URL: www.nia.nih.gov/news/physical-activity-and-alzheimers-related-hippocampal-atrophy. Accessed September 4, 2024.

TIPS FOR HELPING A PERSON WITH DEMENTIA STAY ACTIVE
- Take a walk together each day. Exercise benefits caregivers as well.
- Use exercise videos or check your local TV guide for programs designed to help older adults exercise.
- Dance to music. This can be a fun and engaging way to stay active.
- Be realistic about how much activity you can do at one time. Several short "mini-workouts" may be more manageable.
- Ensure they wear comfortable clothes and shoes that fit well and are suitable for exercise.
- Make sure they drink water or juice after exercise to stay hydrated.

Even if the person has difficulty walking, they may still be able to:
- Do simple tasks around the home, such as sweeping and dusting.
- Use a stationary bike.
- Use soft rubber exercise balls or balloons for stretching or tossing back and forth.
- Use stretching bands.
- Lift weights or household items, such as soup cans.

Physical activity plays a vital role in maintaining brain health and preventing cognitive decline, particularly in individuals at risk for AD. Engaging in regular physical activity can help preserve the size of the hippocampus, a critical brain region for memory, and potentially delay AD-related changes.[2]

---

[2] National Institute on Aging (NIA), "Exercising with Chronic Conditions," National Institutes of Health (NIH), April 3, 2020. Available online. URL: www.nia.nih.gov/health/exercise-and-physical-activity/exercising-chronic-conditions#alzheimers. Accessed September 4, 2024.

Section 4.4 | Light Exercise: A Key to Boosting Memory and Brain Health

HOW MUCH EXERCISE DOES IT TAKE TO BOOST YOUR MEMORY SKILLS?

Possibly a lot less than you might think, according to a study examining the effect of light exercise on memory. In their study of 36 healthy young adults, researchers found surprisingly immediate improvements in memory after just 10 minutes of low-intensity pedaling on a stationary bike. Further testing by the international research team reported that this quick, light workout—comparable in intensity to a short yoga or tai chi session—was associated with heightened activity in the brain's hippocampus. This finding is noteworthy because the hippocampus is known for its role in remembering facts and events.

Brain scans of the participants after the light exercise also revealed stronger connections between the hippocampus and the cerebral cortex, which plays an important role in detailed memory processing. Moreover, the level of heightened connectivity in a person's brain after exercise predicted the degree of their memory improvement.

STUDY DETAILS AND FINDINGS

These results come from the labs of Michael Yassa at the University of California, Irvine, and Hideaki Soya at the University of Tsukuba, Japan. Soya's team had conducted earlier studies in rodents that showed increased activity in the hippocampus and improved performance on tests of spatial memory after a light-intensity run on a controlled treadmill. Interestingly, more intense exercise did not offer the same memory boost.

In the study, partly funded by the National Institutes of Health (NIH) and published in *Proceedings of the National Academy of Sciences*, the researchers extended these earlier findings to humans by combining very light-intensity exercise with computerized memory tests and high-resolution functional magnetic

Fitness and Exercise Sourcebook, Seventh Edition

resonance imaging (fMRI) of the brain. Here is how the study was conducted:
- Participants came in on two separate occasions. During each visit, they either participated in 10 minutes of light-intensity biking or sat quietly on the same bike for 10 minutes.
- The biking regimen was calibrated to 30 percent of each person's maximum rate of oxygen consumption during exercise, meeting the definition of "very light" exercise by the American College of Sports Medicine.
- In another round of testing, participants completed a memory test while researchers captured their brain activity using fMRI.

After each biking session and resting session, participants were administered two computerized tests:
1. For the first test, they were shown 196 different images of everyday objects, such as a coffee cup, flashlight, or eyeglasses, and asked whether each object represented an indoor or outdoor item. This phase was designed merely to hold their attention on the images.
2. In the second test, administered 45 minutes later, participants were shown 256 images of everyday objects and asked whether each photo was new, identical to one seen in the first test, or similar. This test was designed to detect even subtle differences in an individual's memory performance.

Participants made fewer errors on the image recognition test after completing 10 minutes of very light exercise compared to when they only rested on the bike. Similar to the earlier rodent studies, subsequent brain scans showed that improved memory performance was accompanied by increased activity and connectivity in the brain.

FUTURE RESEARCH DIRECTIONS
Many questions remain. For example, the observed benefits of just 10 minutes of very light exercise were seen in healthy young

adults. But will light exercise also help people who already have memory problems? Would longer periods of exercise, possibly at a higher intensity level, offer even greater benefits? The researchers are already exploring these questions.

The NIH is funding several other promising studies and consortia that aim to optimize the health benefits of exercise. A particularly exciting project is the Molecular Transducers of Physical Activity Consortium (MoTrPAC). The MoTrPAC effort will develop a comprehensive map of the molecular changes that occur with physical activity, leading to improved performance of multiple body systems. Although it is well-established that exercise is good for us, the mechanisms by which exercise affects our bodies and enhances physical and mental health are less clear. The MoTrPAC project aims to clarify these processes.

IMPLICATIONS FOR PERSONALIZED EXERCISE RECOMMENDATIONS

One of the most encouraging aspects of this latest study is that it suggests light-intensity exercise, which is accessible to most people, provides real benefits for the brain. As more is learned about the underlying biology of exercise and memory, the goal is to enable doctors, personal trainers, and others interested in enhancing health to make more precise exercise recommendations tailored to the specific needs and abilities of each person.[1]

---

[1] "Study Suggests Light Exercise Helps Memory," National Institutes of Health (NIH), October 2, 2018. Available online. URL: https://directorsblog.nih.gov/2018/10/02/study-suggests-light-exercise-helps-memory. Accessed September 4, 2024.

Chapter 5 | The Role of Physical Activity in Health and Weight Management

HEALTH BENEFITS OF REGULAR PHYSICAL ACTIVITY
Regular physical activity provides both immediate and long-term health benefits. It can improve brain health, strengthen bones and muscles, and enhance one's ability to perform everyday tasks. Physical activity also helps:
- improve sleep quality
- reduce high blood pressure (HBP) and the risk of heart disease and stroke
- reduce the risk of type 2 diabetes
- reduce the risk of several forms of cancer
- reduce arthritis pain and associated disability
- reduce the risk of osteoporosis and falls
- reduce symptoms of depression and anxiety

WEIGHT MANAGEMENT AND PHYSICAL ACTIVITY
Physical activity is crucial if you are trying to lose weight or maintain a healthy weight. Increased physical activity raises the number of calories your body uses for energy. Using calories through physical activity, combined with reducing the calories you consume, creates a calorie deficit that results in weight loss.

While most weight loss occurs from decreasing calorie intake, the only sustainable way to maintain weight loss is to engage in regular physical activity.

Fitness and Exercise Sourcebook, Seventh Edition

RECOMMENDED PHYSICAL ACTIVITY LEVELS FOR HEALTH AND WEIGHT MANAGEMENT

For overall health, adults need at least 150 minutes per week of moderate-intensity aerobic activity. This could be achieved by brisk walking for 22 minutes a day, 30 minutes a day for five days a week, or in any way that fits your schedule. Alternatively, 75 minutes of vigorous-intensity aerobic activity per week, such as swimming laps, is recommended. A combination of moderate- and vigorous-intensity aerobic activities can also be effective. Additionally, adults should engage in muscle-strengthening activities at least two days per week.

To maintain a healthy weight, you may need more than the recommended amount of physical activity each week. The exact amount needed varies greatly from person to person.

To lose weight and keep it off, a high amount of physical activity is necessary unless you also adjust your diet to reduce calorie intake. Achieving and maintaining a healthy weight requires both regular physical activity and healthy eating patterns.

UNDERSTANDING MODERATE- AND VIGOROUS-INTENSITY ACTIVITIES

Moderate-intensity physical activity increases your breathing and heart rate, but you can still carry on a conversation. Examples include:
- walking briskly (a 15-minute mile)
- light yard work (raking or bagging leaves, pushing a lawn mower)
- light snow shoveling
- actively playing with children
- biking at a casual pace

Vigorous-intensity physical activity significantly increases your heart rate and makes it difficult to have a conversation. Examples include:
- jogging or running
- swimming laps
- rollerblading or inline skating at a brisk pace

The Role of Physical Activity in Health and Weight Management

- cross-country skiing
- most competitive sports (e.g., football, basketball, soccer)
- jumping rope

CALORIES BURNED IN MODERATE AND VIGOROUS ACTIVITIES

Tables 5.1 and 5.2 present estimates of calories burned during 30 minutes and 1 hour of both moderate and vigorous physical activities for a person weighing 154 pounds. These activities range from moderate efforts, such as hiking and walking, to more vigorous exercises such as running, swimming, and aerobics, highlighting the varying energy expenditure associated with different levels of physical exertion.[1]

Table 5.1. Calories Used in Moderate Physical Activity

Moderate Physical Activity	Approximate Calories/30 Minutes for a 154 lb Person	Approximate Calories/Hr for a 154 lb Person
Hiking	185	370
Light gardening/Yard work	165	330
Dancing	165	330
Golf (walking and carrying clubs)	165	330
Bicycling (<10 mph)	145	290
Walking (3.5 mph)	140	280
Weight lifting (general light workout)	110	220
Stretching	90	180

---

[1] "Physical Activity and Your Weight and Health," Centers for Disease Control and Prevention (CDC), December 27, 2023. Available online. URL: www.cdc.gov/healthy-weight-growth/physical-activity. Accessed September 4, 2024.

Table 5.2. Calories Used in Vigorous Physical Activity

Vigorous Physical Activity	Approximate Calories/30 Minutes for a 154 lb Person	Approximate Calories/Hr for a 154 lb Person
Running/Jogging (5 mph)	295	590
Bicycling (>10 mph)	295	590
Swimming (slow freestyle laps)	255	510
Aerobics	240	510
Walking (4.5 mph)	230	460
Heavy yard work (chopping wood)	220	440
Weight lifting (vigorous effort)	—	440
Basketball (vigorous)	220	440

MAINTAINING A HEALTHY WEIGHT FOR AGING

Maintaining a healthy weight is crucial for healthy aging. Elevated body mass index (BMI) in older adults can increase the likelihood of developing health issues such as heart disease, HBP, stroke, and diabetes. Losing weight or maintaining a healthy weight can help reduce these risks.

Being underweight also poses health risks. A low BMI may increase the likelihood of developing conditions such as osteoporosis and anemia, and it may hinder recovery from illness or infection.

BALANCING DIET AND PHYSICAL ACTIVITY FOR A HEALTHY WEIGHT

Being active and choosing healthy foods can help you maintain or achieve a healthy weight, boost energy levels, and decrease the risk of other health problems. Aim to consume nutrient-rich foods and engage in at least 150 minutes of physical activity each week.

The energy your body gets from foods and drinks is measured in calories. The number of calories needed each day depends on your activity level and other factors.

The Role of Physical Activity in Health and Weight Management

Visit MyPlate Plan (www.myplate.gov/myplate-plan) to determine your daily calorie needs based on your age, sex, height, weight, and physical activity level.
- To lose weight, increase physical activity or reduce calorie intake.
- To gain weight, increase calorie intake while maintaining a moderate activity level.

TIPS FOR MANAGING WEIGHT
Losing Weight
- Limit portion sizes to control calorie intake.
- Be as physically active as possible.
- Swap out usual foods for healthier alternatives.
- Stay hydrated with water; avoid drinks with added sugars.
- Set specific, realistic goals, such as three 15-minute walks per week.
- If there is a break in your healthy eating or exercise routine, get back on track quickly.
- Keep track of what you eat in a food diary.

Gaining Weight
- Eat more foods with healthy fats, such as avocados and peanut butter.
- If you get full quickly, eat smaller meals more frequently.
- Include nutrient-dense snacks such as nuts, cheese, and dried fruit.
- Dine with friends and family to make meals more enjoyable.
- Stay active to stimulate appetite.[2]

---

[2] National Institute on Aging (NIA), "Maintaining a Healthy Weight," National Institutes of Health (NIH), April 7, 2022. Available online. URL: www.nia.nih.gov/health/healthy-eating-nutrition-and-diet/maintaining-healthy-weight. Accessed September 4, 2024.

Chapter 6 | Myths about Nutrition and Physical Activity

Are you overwhelmed by daily decisions about what to eat, how much to eat, when to eat, and how much physical activity you need to be healthy? If so, do not be discouraged because you are not alone. With so many choices and decisions, it can be hard to know what to do and which information you can trust.

FOOD MYTHS

- **Myth 1.** To lose weight, you have to give up all your favorite foods.
  Fact. You do not have to give up all your favorite foods when you are trying to lose weight. Small amounts of your favorite high-calorie foods can be part of your weight-loss plan. Just remember to keep track of the total calories you take in. To lose weight, you must burn more calories than you consume through food and beverages.

- **Myth 2.** Grain products such as bread, pasta, and rice are fattening. You should avoid them when trying to lose weight.
  Fact. Grains themselves are not necessarily fattening or unhealthy, although substituting whole grains for refined-grain products is healthier and may help you feel fuller. The *Dietary Guidelines for Americans, 2020–2025* recommend consuming grains as part of a healthy eating plan. At least half of the grains you eat should be whole grains. Examples of whole grains include brown rice

and whole-wheat bread, cereal, and pasta. Whole grains provide iron, fiber, and other important nutrients.

- **Myth 3**. Choosing foods that are gluten-free will help you eat healthier.
  Fact. Gluten-free foods are not healthier if you do not have celiac disease or are not sensitive to gluten. Gluten is a protein found in wheat, barley, and rye grains. A healthcare professional may prescribe a gluten-free eating plan to treat people with celiac disease or gluten sensitivity. If you do not have these health problems but avoid gluten anyway, you may miss out on essential vitamins, fiber, and minerals. A gluten-free diet is not a weight-loss diet and is not intended to help you lose weight.

- **Myth 4**. You should avoid all fats if you are trying to be healthy or lose weight.
  Fact. You do not have to avoid all fats if you are trying to improve your health or lose weight. Fat provides essential nutrients and should be an important part of a healthy eating plan. However, because fats have more calories per gram than protein or carbohydrates, you must limit fat intake to avoid extra calories. If you are trying to lose weight, consider eating small amounts of foods with healthy fats, such as avocados, olives, or nuts. You can also replace whole-fat cheese or milk with lower-fat versions.

- **Myth 5**. Dairy products are fattening and unhealthy.
  Fact. Dairy products are an important food group because they provide protein, which your body needs to build muscles and help organs function well, and calcium, which strengthens bones. Most dairy products, such as milk and some yogurts, have added vitamin D to help your body use calcium effectively, as many Americans do not get enough of these nutrients. Dairy products made from fat-free or low-fat milk have fewer calories than those made from whole milk.

- **Myth 6**. "Going vegetarian" will help you lose weight and be healthier.
  Fact. Some research shows that a healthy vegetarian eating plan, consisting mostly of plant-based foods, may be

Myths about Nutrition and Physical Activity

linked to lower levels of obesity, lower blood pressure, and a reduced risk of heart disease. However, going vegetarian will only lead to weight loss if you reduce your total calorie intake. Some vegetarians may choose foods high in sugar, fats, and calories, which could lead to weight gain.

PHYSICAL ACTIVITY MYTHS

- **Myth 1.** Physical activity only counts if you do it for long periods of time.
  Fact. You do not need to be active for long periods to meet the recommended amount of regular physical activity, which is at least 150 minutes, or 2 hours and 30 minutes, of moderate-intensity physical activity each week, according to the *Physical Activity Guidelines for Americans, 2nd edition.* An example of moderate-intensity activity is brisk walking. You can spread these sessions out over the week and even do short, 10-minute spurts of activity three times a day on five or more days a week.

- **Myth 2.** Lifting weights is not a good way to improve your health or lose weight because it will make you "bulk up."
  Fact. Lifting weights or engaging in other activities that help build strong muscles, such as push-ups and some types of yoga, two or three days a week will not bulk you up. Only intense strength training, along with certain genetic factors, can build large muscles. Like other kinds of physical activity, muscle-strengthening activities help improve your health and may also help you control your weight by increasing the amount of energy-burning muscle.

People spend a lot of time sitting: at desks, in cars, and in front of computers, TVs, and other electronic devices. Break up your sitting time by getting up and moving around, even if it is only for 10 minutes at a time. Those minutes will add up over days and weeks.[1]

---

[1] "Some Myths about Nutrition & Physical Activity," National Institute of Diabetes and Digestive and Kidney Diseases (NIDDK), April 2017. Available online. URL: www.niddk.nih.gov/health-information/weight-management/myths-nutrition-physical-activity. Accessed September 5, 2024.

Chapter 7 | Physical Inactivity Trends among Adults 50 Years and Older

Overall, 27.5 percent of adults aged 50 years and older were inactive. Inactivity prevalence significantly increased with age: 25.4 percent for adults aged 50–64 years, 26.9 percent for those aged 65–74 years, and 35.3 percent for those aged 75 years and older. Inactivity prevalence was significantly higher among women, Hispanics, non-Hispanic Blacks, and adults with one or more chronic diseases compared with their counterparts. Inactivity prevalence also significantly increased with decreasing levels of education and increasing body mass index (BMI).

WHAT ARE THE IMPLICATIONS FOR PUBLIC HEALTH PRACTICE?
Despite the many benefits of physical activity, approximately one in four adults aged 50 years and older are inactive. Communities can be designed and enhanced to make it safer and easier for people of all ages and abilities to be physically active.

Table 7.1 displays the prevalence of self-reported physical inactivity among adults aged 50 and older, categorized by sex, age group, race/ethnicity, education, BMI, and region, as reported in the Behavioral Risk Factor Surveillance System. It highlights how inactivity rates vary across different demographic and health factors.

Fitness and Exercise Sourcebook, Seventh Edition

Table 7.1. Self-Reported Prevalence of Inactivity* among Adults 50 Years and Older by Selected Characteristics—Behavioral Risk Factor Surveillance System

Sex	Male	25.5%
	Female	29.4%
Age group (years)	50–64	25.4%
	65–74	26.9%
	>75	35.3%
Race/Ethnicity	White, non-Hispanic	26.2%
	Black, non-Hispanic	33.1%
	Hispanic	32.7%
	Others§	27.1%
Education	Below high school graduate	44.1%
	High school graduate	34.7%
	Some college	24.6%
	College graduate	14.2%
Body mass index (kg/m²)	Underweight/Normal weight	23.1%
	Overweight	24.4%
	Obese	35.8%
Region	Midwest	28.4%
	Northeast	26.6%
	South	30.1%
	West	23.1%

* Inactivity is defined as responding "No" to the following question: "During the past month, other than your regular job, did you participate in any physical activities or exercises such as running, calisthenics, golf, gardening, or walking for exercise?"
§ Other includes Multi-Racial, Asian, Native Hawaiian or Other Pacific Islander, or American Indian, Alaska Native.

Table 7.2 presents the self-reported prevalence of physical inactivity among adults aged 50 and older, categorized by the presence of chronic diseases such as arthritis, cancer, coronary heart disease,

Physical Inactivity Trends among Adults 50 Years and Older

chronic obstructive pulmonary disease (COPD), depressive disorder, diabetes, and stroke. It highlights the increased rates of inactivity among individuals with these chronic conditions compared to those without.

Table 7.2. Self-Reported Prevalence of Inactivity* among Adults 50 Years and Older by Chronic Disease—Behavioral Risk Factor Surveillance System

Arthritis	Yes	33.1%
	No	23.3%
Cancer**	Yes	31.6%
	No	27.0%
Coronary heart disease	Yes	37.2%
	No	26.1%
Chronic obstructive pulmonary disease (COPD)	Yes	44.4%
	No	25.6%
Depressive disorder	Yes	38.0%
	No	25.2%
Diabetes	Yes	38.4%
	No	25.1%
Stroke	Yes	42.9%
	No	26.7%

*Inactivity is defined as responding "No" to the following question: "During the past month, other than your regular job, did you participate in any physical activities or exercises such as running, calisthenics, golf, gardening, or walking for exercise?"
** Excluding skin cancer.

Table 7.3 displays the prevalence of self-reported physical inactivity among adults aged 50 and older across different U.S. states. It provides a state-by-state comparison, illustrating variations in inactivity rates as reported in the Behavioral Risk Factor Surveillance System.[1]

---

[1] "Physical Inactivity among Adults 50 Years and Older," Centers for Disease Control and Prevention (CDC), September 2016. Available online. URL: www.cdc.gov/physicalactivity/inactivity-among-adults-50plus/mmwr-data-highlights.pdf. Accessed September 5, 2024.

Table 7.3. Self-Reported Prevalence of Inactivity* among Adults 50 Years and Older by State—Behavioral Risk Factor Surveillance System

States	Prevalence of Inactivity (%)
Alabama	32.3
Alaska	22.9
Arizona	24.3
Arkansas	38.8
California	24.4
Colorado	17.9
Connecticut	24.4
Delaware	28.7
District of Columbia	25.7
Florida	26.5
Georgia	28.7
Hawaii	23.5
Idaho	21.2
Illinois	27.7
Indiana	30.6
Iowa	28.7
Kansas	29.8
Kentucky	34.8
Louisiana	34.0
Maine	23.9
Maryland	24.9
Massachusetts	23.5
Michigan	29.4
Minnesota	23.8
Mississippi	35.6
Missouri	31.1

Physical Inactivity Trends among Adults 50 Years and Older

Table 7.3. Continued

States	Prevalence of Inactivity (%)
Montana	24.1
Nebraska	25.5
Nevada	27.9
New Hampshire	23.2
New Jersey	25.9
New Mexico	24.8
New York	28.5
North Carolina	27.7
North Dakota	27.3
Ohio	30.2
Oklahoma	34.8
Oregon	20.2
Pennsylvania	27.5
Rhode Island	25.6
South Carolina	29.4
South Dakota	24.4
Tennessee	33.3
Texas	31.4
Utah	19.9
Vermont	22.3
Virginia	28.4
Washington	20.0
West Virginia	33.7
Wisconsin	24.1
Wyoming	26.3

* Inactivity is defined as responding "No" to the following question: "During the past month, other than your regular job, did you participate in any physical activities or exercises such as running, calisthenics, golf, gardening, or walking for exercise?"

Part 2 | Guidelines for Lifelong Physical Fitness

Chapter 8 | **Understanding the Physical Activity Guidelines for Americans**

Being physically active is one of the most important actions that people of all ages can take to improve their health. About $117 billion in annual health-care costs and approximately 10 percent of premature mortality are associated with inadequate physical activity, specifically not meeting the aerobic key guidelines. This second edition of the *Physical Activity Guidelines for Americans* (https://health.gov/sites/default/files/2019-09/Physical_Activity_Guidelines_2nd_edition.pdf) provides science-based guidance to help people aged three years and older improve their health through appropriate physical activity. It builds on the *2008 Guidelines* by incorporating new evidence about additional health benefits, offering greater flexibility in how to achieve those benefits, and highlighting proven strategies to increase physical activity and promote supportive communities. The *Physical Activity Guidelines for Americans* is issued by the U.S. Department of Health and Human Services (HHS) and complements the *Dietary Guidelines for Americans*, a joint effort of HHS and the U.S. Department of Agriculture (USDA). Together, these documents provide comprehensive guidance for the U.S. population on the importance of being physically active and maintaining a healthy diet to promote good health and reduce the risk of chronic diseases.

THE RATIONALE FOR PHYSICAL ACTIVITY GUIDELINES

Extensive scientific evidence supports the recommendation that all Americans engage in regular physical activity to improve overall health and reduce the risk of many health problems. Physical activity exemplifies how lifestyle choices significantly affect health, much like other lifestyle factors such as diet, smoking, and alcohol use. The *Physical Activity Guidelines for Americans* provides information and guidance on the types and amounts of physical activity that offer substantial health benefits. Although the primary audience is policymakers and health professionals, the guidelines are also valuable for the public. The main idea is that regular physical activity over months and years can yield long-term health benefits.

The need for the guidelines is underscored by the critical role of physical activity in the health of Americans, whose current inactivity puts them at unnecessary risk. *Healthy People 2020* set objectives to increase physical activity levels among Americans from 2010 to 2020. Although some improvements have been noted, only 26 percent of men, 19 percent of women, and 20 percent of adolescents report sufficient activity to meet the aerobic and muscle-strengthening guidelines.

DISEASE PREVENTION AND HEALTH PROMOTION

The 2008 Advisory Committee Report and the *2008 Guidelines* focused primarily on the disease prevention benefits of physical activity. The 2018 Scientific Report expanded on this by demonstrating that, in addition to disease prevention, regular physical activity provides other benefits, such as improved sleep, enhanced mood, and better performance of daily tasks. The 2018 report also highlights the immediate benefits of physical activity, not just those accrued over months or years. This broader focus on both disease prevention and health promotion is integrated into the key guidelines for various age groups: children and adolescents, adults, older adults, pregnant or postpartum women, and adults with chronic diseases or disabilities.

Key Benefits of Physical Activity
- **Improved sleep quality.** Regular moderate-to-vigorous physical activity helps adults fall asleep faster, reduces the time spent awake after falling asleep, increases time in deep sleep, and decreases daytime sleepiness.

Understanding the Physical Activity Guidelines for Americans

- **Enhanced quality of life (QOL).** Regular physical activity improves perceived QOL, including physical, mental, and emotional health.
- **Improved physical function.** Physical activity enhances physical function across all ages, helping people perform daily tasks with energy and without undue fatigue. For older adults, this reduces the risk of falls and fall-related injuries, aiding in maintaining independence.
- **Improved cognitive function.** Physical activity may enhance memory, attention, executive function (planning, organizing, controlling emotions), and academic performance among youth.

THE IMPORTANCE OF UNDERSTANDABLE GUIDELINES

The HHS aims to keep the *Physical Activity Guidelines for Americans* clear and understandable while remaining consistent with complex scientific information. Each chapter highlights the key guidelines to ensure that the most crucial information is easily identifiable and disseminated to the public and those involved in promoting physical activity.

TAKING ACTION: INCREASING PHYSICAL ACTIVITY LEVELS IN AMERICANS

Action is needed at individual, community, and societal levels to encourage Americans to become more physically active. Making physical activity a safe and easy choice is essential for increasing participation. Evidence-based strategies—those tested and proven to increase physical activity—are vital for achieving this goal. The 2018 Physical Activity Guidelines Advisory Committee's review shows that effective strategies range from one-on-one or small-group interventions to broader community-level programs, practices, and policies that facilitate physical activity.

Promoting regular physical activity is essential for improving public health and reducing the burden of chronic diseases. The

Physical Activity Guidelines for Americans provides clear guidelines and implement evidence-based strategies to enhance the health and well-being of the U.S. population.[1]

---

[1] Office of Disease Prevention and Health Promotion (ODPHP), "Current Guidelines," U.S. Department of Health and Human Services (HHS), August 24, 2021. Available online. URL: https://health.gov/our-work/nutrition-physical-activity/physical-activity-guidelines/current-guidelines. Accessed September 4, 2024.

Chapter 9 | Physical Fitness for Children

Chapter Contents
Section 9.1—Physical Activity Guidelines and Benefits
　　　for Children 57
Section 9.2—Physical Activity for Preschoolers..........................60
Section 9.3—Physical Education and Physical Activity
　　　in Schools 62
Section 9.4—School Guidelines for Health and Fitness..............65

Section 9.1 | Physical Activity Guidelines and Benefits for Children

CHILD ACTIVITY RECOMMENDATIONS
The amount and types of physical activity recommended vary by a child's age.

Children Aged 3–5
Should be physically active throughout the day for growth and development. Adult caregivers should encourage children to be active when they play, for example, by jumping or riding a tricycle.

Children and Adolescents Aged 6–17
This group needs 60 minutes or more of moderate-to-vigorous intensity physical activity each day, including:
- **Aerobic activity.** Most of the 60 minutes or more daily should be spent doing activities such as walking, running, or anything that makes their hearts beat faster. Vigorous-intensity activities should be included at least three days a week.
- **Muscle-strengthening.** Includes activities such as climbing or doing push-ups, at least three days a week.
- **Bone-strengthening.** Includes activities such as jumping or running, at least three days a week.

Sixty minutes of activity a day may sound like a lot, but do not worry! Your children may already be meeting the recommended physical activity levels. Also, school-based physical activity can help children meet the recommended 60 minutes or more of daily physical activity.

ASSESSING AEROBIC INTENSITY
On a scale of 0–10, where sitting is a 0 and the highest level of physical activity is 10, moderate-intensity activity is 5 or 6. Vigorous-intensity activity is 7 or 8.

Fitness and Exercise Sourcebook, Seventh Edition

When children engage in moderate-intensity activity, their hearts beat faster, and they breathe much harder than when they are at rest or sitting. For example, when children walk to school with friends each morning, they are probably doing moderate-intensity aerobic activity. But when they run or chase others while playing tag during recess, they are likely engaging in vigorous-intensity activity.

AGE-APPROPRIATE ACTIVITIES

Some physical activities are better suited for children than adolescents. For example, younger children usually strengthen their muscles when they do gymnastics, play on a jungle gym, or climb trees.

Children typically do not need formal muscle-strengthening programs, such as weightlifting. As they grow older and become adolescents, they may start structured weightlifting programs. These types of programs can be done alongside their sports team practices.[1]

STRATEGIES TO KEEP YOUR CHILD PHYSICALLY ACTIVE

Physical activities can range from informal, active play to organized sports.
- **Start early.** Young children love to play and be physically active. Encouraging lots of safe and unstructured movement and play can help build a strong foundation for an active lifestyle.
- **Make physical activity fun.** Fun activities can be anything your child enjoys, whether structured or unstructured. Activities can range from team or individual sports to recreational activities, such as walking, running, skating, bicycling, swimming, playground activities, or free-time play.

Here are some ways to do this:
- Make physical activity part of your family's daily routine by taking family walks or playing active games together.
- Give your children equipment that encourages physical activity.

---

[1] "Child Activity: An Overview," Centers for Disease Control and Prevention (CDC), January 8, 2024. Available online. URL: www.cdc.gov/physical-activity-basics/guidelines/children.html. Accessed September 5, 2024.

Physical Fitness for Children

- Take young people to places they can be physically active, such as public parks, community baseball fields, or basketball courts.
- Be positive about the physical activities in which your child participates. Encourage interest in new activities.
- Instead of watching television after dinner, help your child find fun physical activities, such as walking, playing chase, or riding bikes.
- Always provide protective equipment such as helmets, wrist pads, or knee pads for activities such as riding bicycles or scooters, skateboarding, roller skating, and rock-wall climbing. Ensure that activities are appropriate for your child's age.

HELPING YOUR CHILD ACHIEVE PHYSICAL ACTIVITY GOALS

Children and adolescents need aerobic activity, which is anything that makes their hearts beat faster. They also need bone-strengthening activities, such as running or jumping, and muscle-strengthening activities, such as climbing or push-ups. Many physical activities fall under more than one type of activity. This makes it possible for your child to do two or even three types of physical activity in one day! For example:

- If your daughter practices basketball with her team every day, she is doing vigorous-intensity aerobic and bone-strengthening activities.
- If your son takes gymnastics lessons, he is doing vigorous-intensity aerobic, muscle-strengthening, and bone-strengthening activities.

It is easy to fit each type of activity into your child's schedule—all it takes is being familiar with the recommendations and finding physical activities your child enjoys.

School-based physical activity programs can also help children meet the recommended levels of daily physical activity.[2]

---

[2] "Making Physical Activity Part of a Child's Life," Centers for Disease Control and Prevention (CDC), August 7, 2024. Available online. URL: www.cdc.gov/physical-activity-basics/adding-children-adolescents/index.html. Accessed September 5, 2024.

HEALTH BENEFITS OF PHYSICAL ACTIVITY FOR CHILDREN

- Improves attention and memory.
- Reduces risk of depression.
- Builds strong muscles and endurance.
- Improves blood pressure and aerobic fitness.
- Helps maintain normal blood sugar levels, sometimes called "cardiometabolic health."
- Reduces the risk of several chronic diseases, including type 2 diabetes and obesity.
- Strengthens bone.
- Helps regulate body weight and reduce body fat.[3]

Section 9.2 | Physical Activity for Preschoolers

Preschool-aged children (ages three to five years) should be encouraged to move and engage in active play, as well as in structured activities, such as throwing games and bicycle or tricycle riding. To strengthen bones, young children should participate in activities that involve hopping, skipping, jumping, and tumbling. Although the specific amount of activity needed to improve bone health and avoid excess fat in young children is not well-defined, a reasonable target may be three hours per day of activity across all intensities: light, moderate, or vigorous. This is the average amount of activity observed among children of this age and is consistent with guidelines from Canada, the United Kingdom, and the Commonwealth of Australia.[1]

---

[3] "Health Benefits of Physical Activity for Children," Centers for Disease Control and Prevention (CDC), April 3, 2024. Available online. URL: www.cdc.gov/physical-activity-basics/health-benefits/children.html. Accessed September 5, 2024.

[1] Office of Disease Prevention and Health Promotion (ODPHP), "Current Guidelines," U.S. Department of Health and Human Services (HHS), August 24, 2021. Available online. URL: https://health.gov/our-work/nutrition-physical-activity/physical-activity-guidelines/current-guidelines. Accessed September 5, 2024.

Physical Fitness for Children

GUIDELINES FOR PRESCHOOL CHILDREN
Preschool children, aged three to five, should engage in physical activity throughout the day. A reasonable target may be three hours per day of light, moderate, and vigorous-intensity activity.

Adult caregivers should encourage active play that includes different types of activities. This includes unstructured play as well as structured activities, such as throwing games and bicycle or tricycle riding. To strengthen bones, young children should participate in activities that involve hopping, skipping, jumping, and tumbling.[2]

CHILD SAFETY FIRST
As your child becomes more independent, it is important that both you and your child are aware of ways to stay safe. Here are a few tips to protect your child:
- **Explain why it is important to stay out of traffic.** Tell them not to play in the street or run after stray balls.
- **Be cautious when letting your child ride their tricycle.** Keep them on the sidewalk and away from the street, and always have them wear a helmet.
- **Check outdoor playground equipment.** Make sure there are no loose parts or sharp edges.
- **Watch your child at all times, especially when they are playing outside.**
- **Be safe in the water.** Teach your child to swim, but always supervise them when they are in or near any body of water (this includes kiddie pools).
- **Teach your child how to stay safe around strangers.**

HEALTHY BODIES
Here are a few tips to help keep your growing child healthy:
- **Eat meals with your child whenever possible.** Let your child see you enjoying fruits, vegetables, and whole grains at meals and snacks.

---

[2] "Recommendations," National Heart, Lung, and Blood Institute (NHLBI), March 24, 2022. Available online. URL: www.nhlbi.nih.gov/health/heart/physical-activity/tips#Guidelines-for-preschool-children. Accessed September 5, 2024.

- **Ensure your child consumes only a limited amount of food and beverages that contain added sugars, solid fats, or salt.**
- **Provide your child with age-appropriate play equipment, such as balls and plastic bats, but let your preschooler choose what to play.** This makes being active fun for your child.
- **Make sure your child gets the recommended amount of sleep each night.** 10–13 hours per 24 hours (including naps) for preschoolers aged three to five years.[3]

Section 9.3 | Physical Education and Physical Activity in Schools

Physical education is the foundation of a Comprehensive School Physical Activity Program. It is an academic subject characterized by a planned, sequential K–12 curriculum based on the national standards for physical education. Physical education provides cognitive content and instruction designed to develop motor skills, knowledge, and behaviors for physical activity and physical fitness. Supporting schools in establishing daily physical education can provide students with the ability and confidence to be physically active for a lifetime.

There are many benefits of physical education in schools. When students participate in physical education, they can:
- increase their level of physical activity
- improve their grades and standardized test scores
- stay on-task in the classroom

---

[3] "Positive Parenting Tips: Preschoolers (3–5 Years Old)," Centers for Disease Control and Prevention (CDC), May 16, 2024. Available online. URL: www.cdc.gov/child-development/positive-parenting-tips/preschooler-3-5-years.html. Accessed September 5, 2024.

Increased time spent in physical education does not negatively affect students' academic achievement.[1]

SCHOOL-BASED PHYSICAL ACTIVITY IMPROVES HEALTHY AND SUPPORTIVE SCHOOL ENVIRONMENTS

The social and emotional climate (SEC) includes aspects of students' educational experiences that influence their social and emotional development. A positive SEC helps create safe and supportive learning environments that can influence students' engagement in school activities, relationships with peers, staff, family, and the community, as well as their academic performance.

School physical activity policies and practices contribute to the overall SEC and can also help develop students' social and emotional learning (SEL). A Comprehensive School Physical Activity Program (CSPAP) can increase physical activity opportunities before, during, and after school. Offering physical activity programs before and after school and integrating physical activity into classroom time can increase opportunities for social interaction and enjoyment of learning alongside peers.

Schools are in a unique position, regardless of learning mode, to help students attain the recommended 60 minutes of moderate-to-vigorous physical activity daily. Schools can support a CSPAP and reinforce SEL core competencies at the same time.

Strengthening the Link between Physical Activity and Social-Emotional Development in Schools

School leaders can take several actions to promote physical activity and well-being in their schools, including the following:
- Recognize the value of physical education and physical activity for health, enjoyment, challenge, self-expression, and social interaction.
- Support physical activity integration in the classroom to reinforce what is taught in physical education and give students a chance to practice their new knowledge and skills.

---

[1] "Physical Education," Centers for Disease Control and Prevention (CDC), July 26, 2022. Available online. URL: www.cdc.gov/healthyschools/physicalactivity/physical-education.htm. Accessed September 5, 2024.

- Offer daily recess for free play and socialization, which are important for building connections with other students.
- Encourage teachers and staff to model active lifestyles and strengthen relationships with students by being physically active during the school day.
- Promote equitable access to physical activity by communicating to parents, teachers, and staff about free and low-cost activities that can be done at home and resources in the community that do not require extra equipment or facilities.
- Partner with local government to create shared-use agreements to allow public access to school facilities, such as gymnasiums, playgrounds, running tracks, and sports fields.
- Implement policies that prohibit using physical activity as punishment (e.g., running laps) or withholding opportunities for physical activity as punishment (e.g., not allowing students to participate in recess).

Cultivating a Positive Social and Emotional Climate through Physical Activity and Social and Emotional Learning in Schools

Examples of actions to support this effort include:
- assessing physical education and physical activity policies and practices for alignment with SEC principles and SEL core competencies
- incorporating SEC and SEL into existing policies (e.g., Comprehensive School Physical Activity Program, local school wellness policy) and school improvement plans
- using physical education content, active classroom strategies, and recess practices that align with SEL core competencies
- communicating with parents about the connections between physical activity, SEC, and SEL, including benefits for students' health and academic success[2]

---

[2] "School-Based Physical Activity Improves Healthy and Supportive School Environments," Centers for Disease Control and Prevention (CDC), July 27, 2022. Available online. URL: www.cdc.gov/healthyschools/school_based_pa_se_sel.htm. Accessed September 5, 2024.

Physical Fitness for Children

Section 9.4 | School Guidelines for Health and Fitness

The Centers for Disease Control and Prevention (CDC) has integrated research and best practices related to promoting healthy eating and physical activity in schools, culminating in the School Health Guidelines. These nine guidelines provide a foundation for developing, implementing, and evaluating school-based policies and practices that encourage healthy eating and physical activity for students.

USE A COORDINATED APPROACH TO DEVELOP, IMPLEMENT, AND EVALUATE HEALTHY EATING AND PHYSICAL ACTIVITY POLICIES AND PRACTICES

Representatives from different segments of the school and community, including parents and students, should work together to maximize healthy eating and physical activity opportunities for students.
- Coordinate healthy eating and physical activity policies through a school health council and school health coordinator.
- Assess current healthy eating and physical activity policies and practices.
- Develop, implement, and monitor these policies systematically.
- Evaluate the effectiveness of the policies and practices regularly.

ESTABLISH SCHOOL ENVIRONMENTS THAT SUPPORT HEALTHY EATING AND PHYSICAL ACTIVITY

The school environment should encourage all students to make healthy eating choices and be physically active throughout the school day.
- Provide access to healthy foods, physical activity opportunities, and safe spaces for these activities.
- Foster a climate that encourages healthy behaviors and does not stigmatize students.
- Promote a healthy body image, acceptance of diverse abilities, and a no-tolerance policy for weight-based teasing.

PROVIDE A QUALITY SCHOOL MEAL PROGRAM AND ENSURE HEALTHY FOOD AND BEVERAGE CHOICES OUTSIDE THE PROGRAM

Schools should model and reinforce healthy dietary behaviors by offering nutritious and appealing foods and beverages in all food venues within the school, including school meals, vending machines, and during events and programs.

- Promote access to and participation in nutritious school meals.
- Ensure all foods and beverages provided are nutritious and appealing.
- Adhere to the Dietary Guidelines for Americans in all food service offerings.

IMPLEMENT A COMPREHENSIVE PHYSICAL ACTIVITY PROGRAM WITH QUALITY PHYSICAL EDUCATION AS THE CORNERSTONE

Children and adolescents should engage in at least 60 minutes of physical activity daily. Schools should offer a comprehensive, school-based physical activity program that includes physical education, recess, classroom activities, and extracurricular activities.

- Provide daily physical education for all students, using a curriculum consistent with national or state standards.
- Provide a significant portion of the daily recommended physical activity through physical education classes.
- Use instructional strategies that build students' skills, confidence, and motivation to stay active.
- Offer ample opportunities for physical activity outside of physical education classes.

IMPLEMENT HEALTH EDUCATION THAT PROVIDES STUDENTS WITH THE KNOWLEDGE AND SKILLS NEEDED FOR LIFELONG HEALTHY EATING AND PHYSICAL ACTIVITY

Health education is crucial for equipping students with the knowledge and skills to lead healthy lives.

- Implement health education from pre-kindergarten through grade 12.

Physical Fitness for Children

- Implement a sequential, culturally appropriate health education curriculum based on national standards.
- Use evidence-based curricula that promote healthy eating and physical activity behaviors.
- Engage students through interactive, relevant instructional methods.

PROVIDE STUDENTS WITH HEALTH, MENTAL HEALTH, AND SOCIAL SERVICES TO ADDRESS HEALTHY EATING, PHYSICAL ACTIVITY, AND RELATED CHRONIC DISEASE PREVENTION

Schools play a role in the physical, mental, and social health of students, providing resources for the identification, treatment, and follow-up of health and mental health conditions related to diet and physical activity.

- Assess and address student needs related to physical activity, nutrition, and obesity.
- Ensure access to health, mental health, and social services.
- Advocate for and coordinate effective school physical activity and nutrition policies.

PARTNER WITH FAMILIES AND COMMUNITY MEMBERS TO DEVELOP AND IMPLEMENT HEALTHY EATING AND PHYSICAL ACTIVITY PROGRAMS

Collaboration with families and community members enhances student learning, promotes consistent health messaging, and increases resources.

- Promote communication between schools, families, and community members to support healthy behaviors.
- Involve families and community members in school health councils.
- Motivate families to participate in programs promoting healthy eating and physical activity.
- Utilize community resources to provide opportunities for healthy eating and physical activity.

PROVIDE A SCHOOL EMPLOYEE WELLNESS PROGRAM THAT INCLUDES HEALTHY EATING AND PHYSICAL ACTIVITY SERVICES

Employee wellness programs can improve staff productivity, reduce absenteeism, and lower health-care costs.
- Assess the nutrition and physical activity needs of school staff.
- Encourage administrative support for employee wellness initiatives.
- Develop and evaluate wellness programs focusing on healthy eating and physical activity.

EMPLOY QUALIFIED STAFF AND PROVIDE PROFESSIONAL DEVELOPMENT OPPORTUNITIES

Hiring certified and qualified staff and offering professional development opportunities ensures quality education and services.
- Hire certified and well-prepared physical education teachers, health education teachers, and nutrition services staff.
- Offer annual professional development for school staff involved in physical education, health education, and nutrition services.
- Provide training for health, mental health, and social services staff, as well as those overseeing extracurricular activities and meal times.[1]

---

[1] "School Health Guidelines," Centers for Disease Control and Prevention (CDC), February 15, 2021. Available online. URL: www.cdc.gov/healthyschools/npao/strategies.htm. Accessed September 6, 2024.

Chapter 10 | **Physical Fitness for Teenagers**

As you grow up, you start making more choices that affect your body and health. Picking healthy foods and drinks, staying active, and getting enough sleep are important for both your physical and mental well-being. These choices can help you:
- have more energy
- build strong bones and muscles
- reach and stay at a healthy weight
- perform better in school
- lower your risk of developing weight-related health problems—both now and as you age

HOW DOES MY BODY USE ENERGY?
Energy is essential for growth. The calories you get from foods and drinks provide that energy. How many calories you need each day depends on various factors, including:
- your age, sex, height, and weight
- how much you are still growing
- how physically active you are

WHAT FOODS AND BEVERAGES SHOULD I CHOOSE?
Your healthy eating plan should include a variety of foods and drinks that are high in nutrients such as vitamins, minerals, fiber, lean protein, complex carbohydrates, and healthy fats. Try to choose foods and beverages that are low in saturated fats, added sugars, and sodium, a mineral found in table salt and in many packaged or prepared foods.

Fitness and Exercise Sourcebook, Seventh Edition

HOW MUCH PHYSICAL ACTIVITY DO I NEED?
Physical activity should be part of your daily life, whether through playing sports, taking physical education (P.E.) classes in school, doing chores, or getting around by biking or public transportation. Even taking a walk can be great for your health if you can do so safely. The benefits of regular physical activity include:
- improved health
- stronger bones and muscles
- reaching and maintaining a healthy weight
- better thinking, mood, and school performance
- lower risk of developing many health problems, such as obesity, diabetes, and heart disease

Current physical activity guidelines recommend that teens engage in at least 60 minutes of physical activity every day, including:
- aerobic activities on most days, which can be either moderate- or vigorous-intensity, such as jogging, biking, or dancing
- activities that strengthen muscles, such as weightlifting or push-ups, at least three days a week
- activities that strengthen bones, such as jumping rope or playing basketball, at least three days a week

You do not have to complete your 60 minutes of activity all at once. Here are some ways to fit it into your day:
- **In the morning**. Try walking to the bus stop or to school.
- **At school**. Be active with friends in P.E. classes, sports, or other activities.
- **After school**. Join a sports team or take your dog for a walk.

HOW CAN I ADD MORE PHYSICAL ACTIVITY TO MY DAY?
Spend Time Away from Your Phone and Other Screens
Teens spend much of their day sitting in classes or doing homework. Spending additional time on your smartphone, watching TV, or playing video games can lead to even more hours of inactivity.

Physical Fitness for Teenagers

Try to limit your screen time to less than two hours each day, not counting time spent on homework or after-school jobs.

Be Active with Friends and Family Members
Being active can be more fun with friends and family members.
- Join a sports team or dance club to be more active and make new friends.
- Challenge your friends and family members to be healthy with you. When they are available, sign up for activities together, such as charity walks, fun runs, or scavenger hunts.
- Do activities that get you moving, such as walking around a park or your neighborhood.
- Have fun outdoors playing basketball, soccer, or flag football.
- Mix things up by choosing a different activity each day.

Try Free or Low-Cost Options
You do not need money or expensive equipment to stay active.
- You can run and use free community facilities, such as school tracks and basketball courts.
- If you want to play a sport or game that requires equipment, check with neighbors or friends at school to see if you can borrow or share supplies.
- If you are interested in joining a sports team, ask your school guidance counselor or a P.E. teacher or coach about costs. They may know if your school waives or reduces fees or if you could apply for a scholarship for certain activities.
- Look for dance and other fitness and exercise videos at your local library, online, on social media, or on some TV channels. If you have a gaming system, check out active sports games.

Keep Moving
Routine chores, such as cleaning your room or taking out the trash, may not elevate your heart rate the way biking and running do, but

they keep you moving. Fitness apps that you can download onto your computer, smartphone, or other mobile device can help you keep track of how active you are each day.

HOW MUCH SLEEP DO I NEED?

Like healthy eating and enough physical activity, getting enough sleep is essential to physical and mental health. You need sufficient sleep to do well at school and work, drive safely, and fight off infection. Not getting enough sleep may also affect your mood and decision-making ability and can lead to gaining excess weight.

Teens should aim for 8–10 hours of sleep each night. Sometimes it is hard to get enough sleep, especially if you have a job, help take care of younger siblings, share a bedroom with others, or are busy with after-school activities. Developing healthy sleeping habits can help. If you can, try to:

- Go to bed and wake up at the same time every day.
- Spend time outside every day.
- Avoid heavy meals within a few hours of bedtime.
- Avoid watching TV or using your computer or smartphone one hour before bedtime.[1]

---

[1] "Take Charge of Your Health: A Guide for Teenagers," National Institute of Diabetes and Digestive and Kidney Diseases (NIDDK), May 2023. Available online. URL: www.niddk.nih.gov/health-information/weight-management/take-charge-health-guide-teenagers. Accessed September 6, 2024.

Chapter 11 | Promoting Physical Activity in Youth

Chapter Contents
Section 11.1—Physical Activity Guidelines for Children and
 Adolescents 75
Section 11.2—The Role of Physical Activity in Youth Health
 and Academic Success 79
Section 11.3—Benefits of Physical Activity for Girls 81
Section 11.4—Balancing Screen Time and Physical Activity
 for a Healthy Lifestyle 83

Section 11.1 | Physical Activity Guidelines for Children and Adolescents

PROMOTING PHYSICAL ACTIVITY FOR LIFELONG HEALTH IN CHILDREN AND ADOLESCENTS

Childhood and adolescence are critical periods for developing movement skills, learning healthy habits, and establishing a foundation for lifelong health and well-being. Regular physical activity in children and adolescents promotes health and fitness. Compared to those who are inactive, physically active youth have higher levels of cardiorespiratory fitness and stronger muscles. They also typically have lower body fat and stronger bones. Physical activity has brain health benefits for school-aged children, including improved cognition and reduced symptoms of depression. Evidence indicates that both acute bouts and regular moderate-to-vigorous physical activity improve cognitive functions such as memory, executive function, processing speed, attention, and academic performance.

Youth who are regularly active have a better chance of a healthy adulthood. Children and adolescents typically do not develop chronic diseases, such as heart disease, hypertension, type 2 diabetes, or osteoporosis. However, current evidence shows that obesity and other risk factors for these diseases, such as elevated insulin, blood lipids, and blood pressure, are increasingly appearing in children and adolescents. Exercise training in youth with overweight or obesity can improve body composition by reducing overall levels of body fat as well as abdominal fat. Regular physical activity also makes it less likely that these risk factors will develop and more likely that children remain healthy into adulthood.

School-aged youth (ages 6–17 years) can achieve substantial health benefits by doing moderate- and vigorous-intensity physical activity for periods that add up to 60 minutes or more each day. This activity should include aerobic activity as well as age-appropriate muscle- and bone-strengthening activities. As with adults, the total amount of physical activity is more important for achieving health benefits than any single component (frequency, intensity, or duration) or specific mix of activities (aerobic, muscle strengthening, bone strengthening). Even so, bone-strengthening activities remain especially important for children and young adolescents because the greatest gains in bone mass occur during the years just before and during puberty. In addition, the majority of peak bone mass is obtained by the end of adolescence.

Parents and other adults who work with or care for youth should be familiar with the key guidelines in this chapter. Adults play an important role in providing age-appropriate opportunities for physical activity. By doing so, they help lay a foundation for lifelong, health-promoting physical activity. Adults need to encourage active play and sustained, structured activity in children as they grow older. As children become adolescents, they typically reduce their physical activity, making it all the more important for adults to provide age-appropriate, enjoyable opportunities for physical activity and to encourage participation.

KEY GUIDELINES FOR SCHOOL-AGED CHILDREN AND ADOLESCENTS

It is important to provide young people with opportunities and encouragement to participate in physical activities that are appropriate for their age, are enjoyable, and offer variety.

Children and adolescents aged 6–17 years should do 60 minutes (1 hour) or more of moderate-to-vigorous physical activity daily:
- **Aerobic**. Most of the 60 minutes or more per day should consist of moderate- or vigorous-intensity aerobic physical activity and should include vigorous-intensity physical activity on at least 3 days a week.
- **Muscle-strengthening**. As part of their 60 minutes or more of daily physical activity, children and adolescents should include muscle-strengthening physical activity on at least 3 days a week.
- **Bone-strengthening**. As part of their 60 minutes or more of daily physical activity, children and adolescents should include bone-strengthening physical activity on at least 3 days a week.

AGE-APPROPRIATE PHYSICAL ACTIVITY GUIDELINES FOR CHILDREN AND ADOLESCENTS

Children and adolescents should meet the key guidelines by doing activities that are appropriate for their age. Their natural patterns of movement differ from those of adults. For example, children are naturally active in an intermittent way, particularly during unstructured active play. During recess and in their free play and games, children engage in basic aerobic and bone-strengthening activities such as running, hopping, skipping, and jumping to develop movement patterns and skills. They alternate brief periods of moderate- and vigorous-intensity activity with periods of light-intensity physical activity or rest. Any episode of moderate- or vigorous-intensity physical activity, however brief, counts toward the key guidelines for children and adolescents aged 6–17 years. For preschool-aged children, activity of any intensity counts, including light intensity.

Children commonly increase muscle strength through unstructured activities that involve lifting or moving their body weight or working against resistance. They typically do not need formal muscle-strengthening programs, such as lifting weights. However, these programs are safe for children if they are properly prescribed and supervised.

As children grow into adolescents, their patterns of physical activity change. They are able to play organized games and sports and sustain longer periods of activity. However, they still commonly engage in intermittent activity, and any period of moderate- or vigorous-intensity activity can count toward the key guidelines.

During the transition to adolescence, sex differences in physical activity behavior appear. The amount of physical activity done by girls tends to decrease dramatically compared to boys, and this disparity persists into adulthood. Therefore, adolescent girls may need additional support and encouragement to maintain health-enhancing physical activity.

Adolescents may meet the key guidelines by engaging in free play, sports, or structured programs. Structured exercise programs can include muscle-strengthening activities, such as lifting weights, working with resistance bands, or using body weight for resistance (such as push-ups, pull-ups, and planks). Muscle-strengthening activities count if they involve a moderate or greater level of effort

Fitness and Exercise Sourcebook, Seventh Edition

and work the major muscle groups of the body—legs, hips, back, abdomen, chest, shoulders, and arms.

Table 11.1 provides examples of physical activities that promote aerobic, muscle-strengthening, and bone-strengthening benefits for both school-aged children and adolescents. Activities are categorized by moderate- and vigorous-intensity aerobic exercises, muscle-strengthening activities, and bone-strengthening exercises, showcasing a variety of ways to engage in physical fitness across different age groups.[1]

Table 11.1. Examples of Aerobic, Muscle-, and Bone-Strengthening Physical Activities for Children and Adolescents

Type of Physical Activity	School-Aged Children	Adolescents
Moderate-intensity aerobic	• Brisk walking • Bicycle riding • Active recreation, such as hiking, riding a scooter without a motor, swimming • Playing games that require catching and throwing, such as baseball and softball	• Brisk walking • Bicycle riding • Active recreation, such as kayaking, hiking, swimming • Playing games that require catching and throwing, such as baseball and softball • House and yard work, such as sweeping or pushing a lawn mower • Some video games that include continuous movement
Vigorous-intensity aerobic	• Running • Bicycle riding • Active games involving running and chasing, such as tag or flag football • Jumping rope • Cross-country skiing • Sports such as soccer, basketball, swimming, tennis • Martial arts • Vigorous dancing	• Running • Bicycle riding • Active games involving running and chasing, such as flag football • Jumping rope • Cross-country skiing • Sports such as soccer, basketball, swimming, tennis • Martial arts • Vigorous dancing

[1] Office of Disease Prevention and Health Promotion (ODPHP), "Current Guidelines," U.S. Department of Health and Human Services (HHS), August 24, 2021. Available online. URL: https://health.gov/our-work/nutrition-physical-activity/physical-activity-guidelines/current-guidelines. Accessed September 4, 2024.

Table 11.1. Continued

Type of Physical Activity	School-Aged Children	Adolescents
Muscle strengthening	• Games such as tug of war • Resistance exercises using body weight or resistance bands • Rope or tree climbing • Climbing on playground equipment • Some forms of yoga	• Games such as tug of war • Resistance exercises using body weight, resistance bands, weight machines, hand-held weights • Some forms of yoga
Bone strengthening	• Hopping, skipping, jumping • Jumping rope • Running • Sports that involve jumping or rapid change in direction	• Jumping rope • Running • Sports that involve jumping or rapid change in direction

Section 11.2 | The Role of Physical Activity in Youth Health and Academic Success

The *Physical Activity Guidelines for Americans, 2nd edition* recommends that children and adolescents aged 6–17 years engage in 60 minutes or more of moderate-to-vigorous physical activity daily.

BENEFITS OF PHYSICAL ACTIVITY

Regular physical activity can help children and adolescents improve cardiorespiratory fitness, build strong bones and muscles, control weight, reduce symptoms of anxiety and depression, and lower the risk of developing health conditions such as:
- heart disease
- cancer
- type 2 diabetes
- high blood pressure (HBP)
- osteoporosis
- obesity

CONSEQUENCES OF PHYSICAL INACTIVITY
Physical inactivity can:
- lead to energy imbalance, such as expending less energy through physical activity than consumed through diet, which can increase the risk of becoming overweight or obese
- increase the risk of factors for cardiovascular disease, including hyperlipidemia (e.g., high cholesterol and triglyceride levels), HBP, obesity, insulin resistance, and glucose intolerance
- increase the risk of developing type 2 diabetes
- increase the risk of developing breast, colon, endometrial, and lung cancers
- lead to low bone density, which in turn leads to osteoporosis

PHYSICAL ACTIVITY BEHAVIORS OF YOUNG PEOPLE
- Less than one-quarter (24 percent) of children aged 6–17 years participate in 60 minutes of physical activity every day.
- In 2017, only 26.1 percent of high school students participated in at least 60 minutes per day of physical activity on all seven days of the previous week.
- In 2017, 51.1 percent of high school students participated in muscle-strengthening exercises, such as push-ups, sit-ups, or weight lifting, on three or more days during the previous week.
- In 2017, 51.7 percent of high school students attended physical education classes on average weekly, but only 29.9 percent attended these classes daily.

RECOMMENDATIONS FOR PHYSICAL ACTIVITY
- **Aerobic.** Most of the 60 minutes or more per day should be either moderate—or vigorous-intensity aerobic physical activity, and vigorous-intensity physical activity should be included at least three days a week.

Promoting Physical Activity in Youth

- **Muscle-strengthening.** Children and adolescents should include muscle-strengthening physical activity at least three days a week as part of their 60 minutes or more of daily physical activity.
- **Bone-strengthening.** Children and adolescents should include bone-strengthening physical activity at least three days a week as part of their 60 minutes or more of daily physical activity.

These guidelines state that children and adolescents should be provided opportunities and encouragement to participate in physical activities that are age-appropriate, enjoyable, and offer variety.

PHYSICAL ACTIVITY AND ACADEMIC ACHIEVEMENT

Students who are physically active tend to have better grades, school attendance, cognitive performance (such as memory), and classroom behaviors (such as on-task behavior).

Higher physical activity and physical fitness levels are associated with improved cognitive performance, including better concentration and memory, among students.[1]

Section 11.3 | Benefits of Physical Activity for Girls

You may wonder if being physically active is really worth the time and effort. Many girls think so! They know that being active is a great way to have fun and spend time with friends. Plus, staying fit can do amazing things for both your mind and body.

---

[1] "Physical Activity Facts," Centers for Disease Control and Prevention (CDC), July 26, 2022. Available online. URL: www.cdc.gov/healthyschools/physicalactivity/facts.htm. Accessed September 3, 2024.

MENTAL HEALTH

Did you know that being physically active can affect how good you feel? It can also affect how well you perform tasks and how pleasant you are to be around. This is partly because physical activity prompts your brain to produce "feel-good" chemicals called "endorphins." Regular physical activity may help you by:
- reducing stress
- improving sleep
- boosting your energy
- reducing symptoms of anxiety and depression
- increasing your self-esteem
- making you feel proud for taking good care of yourself
- improving how well you perform at school

OVERALL HEALTH

Being physically active is great for your muscles, heart, and lungs. It may even help with unpleasant premenstrual syndrome (PMS) symptoms! Some other possible benefits of the activity include:
- **Building strong bones**. Your body creates the most bone when you are a kid and a teen. You can learn more about how to build strong bones.
- **Promoting a healthy weight**. Obesity is a serious problem among kids in the United States. It can lead to problems with your sleep, knees, heart, emotions, and more, but exercise can help.
- **Helping prevent diabetes**. A growing number of young people are developing diabetes. Regular physical activity can help prevent one type of diabetes.
- **Building healthy habits**. If you get used to being active now, you are more likely to continue when you are older. You will thank yourself later!
- **Fighting cancer**. Research shows that exercise may help protect against certain kinds of cancer, including breast cancer.
- **Helping prevent high blood pressure (HBP)**. The number of kids with HBP is increasing. HBP makes

your heart and arteries work harder to pump blood and increases the risk of conditions such as kidney and eye diseases.

Are you worried that exercise will bulk you up? Exercising will not give you big, bulging muscles—it takes a very intense weight-lifting program to achieve a bodybuilder's look. Exercise and other forms of physical activity can help if you need to lose weight or want to maintain a healthy weight.[1]

Section 11.4 | Balancing Screen Time and Physical Activity for a Healthy Lifestyle

ENCOURAGING FAMILY ACTIVITIES FOR A HEALTHY WEIGHT

Whether it is taking a family walk on a Saturday morning or after dinner, or washing the car together, everyone is encouraged to get active to maintain a healthy weight.

By getting active, you are using calories stored from everything consumed throughout the day. Everything your family eats and drinks (from breakfast to dinner) is stored as energy. If this stored energy is not used, it creates an imbalance that can lead to weight gain.

However, balancing food intake and activity is possible. When discussing moving more, the goal is not to train like athletes. Some types of physical activity and exercise burn significant energy, but everyday activities use energy, too. For example, simply parking farther away from the grocery store and walking the extra distance can use more energy.

It is up to each individual to choose the activities that are right for them and their family. It is also essential to stick with it. It is easy to spend a lot of time sitting in front of the computer or television (TV).

---

[1] girlshealth.gov, "Why Physical Activity Is Important," Office on Women's Health (OWH), June 22, 2015. Available online. URL: www.girlshealth.gov/fitness/whygetfit. Accessed September 5, 2024.

The same is true for children. They spend hours sitting at school, at home doing homework, and in front of the TV or computer.

LIMIT COMPUTER TIME AND TELEVISION USAGE

For many, limiting computer use and getting away from screens can be challenging. "Screen time" refers to TV screens, computer monitors, and even handheld devices used for checking email, listening to music, watching TV, and playing video games.

Health experts recommend limiting screen time at home to two hours or less each day. Time spent in front of the screen, unless work- or homework-related, could be better spent engaging in physical activity (increasing energy output).

As a parent or caregiver, set a good example for children by establishing rules that limit computer time, TV watching, and video game playing. Research by the Henry J. Kaiser Foundation shows that setting rules about media use is difficult for many parents.

In 8- to 18-year-olds:
- 28 percent said their parents set TV-watching rules
- 30 percent said their parents set rules about video game use
- 36 percent said their parents set rules about computer use

However, the same study also showed that when parents set media rules, children's media use was almost three hours lower per day.

TIPS TO REDUCE SCREEN TIME
Talk to Your Family
Explain to your children the importance of sitting less and moving more to stay healthy. Tell them they will have more energy, and it will help them develop or improve skills such as riding a bike or shooting hoops, leading to more fun with friends. Let them know you will do the same.

Set a Good Example
Be a good role model by limiting your screen time to no more than two hours per day. If your children see you following the rules, they will be more likely to do the same.

Log Screen Time versus Active Time
Track how much time your family spends in front of screens, including TV watching, playing video games, and using the computer for non-work or non-school activities. Then compare that to how much physical activity they are getting. This will help you understand what changes may be needed.

Make Screen Time = Active Time
When spending time in front of a screen, do something active. Stretch, do yoga, or lift weights. You can also challenge the family to see who can do the most push-ups, jumping jacks, or leg lifts during TV commercial breaks.

Set Screen Time Limits
Create a household rule that limits screen time to two hours every day. More importantly, enforce the rule.

Create Screen-Free Bedrooms
Do not put a TV or computer in your child's bedroom. Children with TVs in their rooms tend to watch about 1.5 hours more TV daily than those without TVs. Additionally, keeping the TV out of their room encourages more family time.

Make Meal Time = Family Time
Turn off the TV during meals. Better yet, remove the TV from the eating area if there is one there. Family meals are a good time to talk. Research shows that families who eat together tend to consume more nutritious meals. Make eating together a priority and schedule family meals at least two to three times a week.

Provide Other Options
Watching TV can become a habit, making it easy to forget about other activities. Offer your children alternatives, such as playing outside, getting a new hobby, or learning a sport.

Do Not Use TV Time as a Reward or Punishment
Using TV as a reward or punishment makes it seem even more important to children.[1]

---

[1] "Reduce Screen Time," National Heart, Lung, and Blood Institute (NHLBI), February 13, 2013. Available online. URL: www.nhlbi.nih.gov/health/educational/wecan/reduce-screen-time/index.htm. Accessed September 6, 2024.

Chapter 12 | Physical Fitness for Adults

Chapter Contents
Section 12.1—Key Guidelines for Physical Activity in Adults...89
Section 12.2—Preventing Heart Disease in Women through
 Physical Activity..93
Section 12.3—Physical Activity during Pregnancy and
 Postpartum...96
Section 12.4—Physical Activity and the Menstrual Cycle..........99
Section 12.5—Managing Weight and Health through
 Physical Activity..101

Section 12.1 | Key Guidelines for Physical Activity in Adults

Adults who are physically active are healthier, feel better, and are less likely to develop chronic diseases such as cardiovascular disease, type 2 diabetes, and several types of cancer compared to inactive adults. Regular moderate-to-vigorous physical activity also reduces feelings of anxiety and depression and improves sleep and quality of life (QOL). Even a single episode of physical activity can temporarily improve cognitive function and reduce anxiety. Physically active adults are better able to perform everyday tasks without undue fatigue. Increased amounts of moderate-to-vigorous physical activity are associated with improved cardiorespiratory and muscular fitness, including healthier body weight and composition. Adults who are more physically active can more easily carry out daily tasks such as climbing stairs, carrying heavy packages, and performing household chores. These benefits apply to men and women of all ages, races, and ethnicities.

Adults gain most of these health benefits when they do the equivalent of 150–300 minutes of moderate-intensity aerobic physical activity each week. Adults gain additional and more extensive health benefits with even more physical activity. Muscle-strengthening activities also provide health benefits and are an important part of an adult's overall physical activity plan.

KEY GUIDELINES FOR ADULTS
- Adults should move more and sit less throughout the day. Some physical activity is better than none. Adults who sit less and engage in any amount of moderate-to-vigorous physical activity gain health benefits.
- For substantial health benefits, adults should engage in at least 150–300 minutes per week of moderate-intensity aerobic physical activity, 75–150 minutes per week of vigorous-intensity aerobic physical activity, or an equivalent combination of both. Aerobic activity should preferably be spread throughout the week.

- Engaging in physical activity beyond the equivalent of 300 minutes of moderate-intensity physical activity a week can provide additional health benefits.
- Adults should also do muscle-strengthening activities of moderate or greater intensity that involve all major muscle groups on two or more days a week, as these activities provide additional health benefits.

AEROBIC ACTIVITY

Aerobic activities, also called "endurance" or "cardio activities," involve moving large muscles in a rhythmic manner for a sustained period. Running, brisk walking, bicycling, playing basketball, dancing, and swimming are all examples of aerobic activities. Aerobic activity increases heart rate and breathing to meet the demands of movement. Over time, regular aerobic activity improves the strength and fitness of the cardiorespiratory system.

The purpose of aerobic activity does not affect whether it counts toward meeting the key guidelines. Physical activity performed during work or as active transportation (such as walking or bicycling) can count as long as the intensity is sufficient. For health benefits, the total amount of moderate-to-vigorous physical activity is more important than the length of each activity episode.

How Much Total Activity Is Recommended Each Week?

When adults engage in at least 150 minutes of moderate-intensity aerobic activity each week, the benefits are substantial. These include lower risks of all-cause mortality, coronary heart disease, stroke, hypertension, type 2 diabetes, certain cancers, anxiety, depression, and Alzheimer disease (AD) and other dementias. Physically active adults also sleep better, have improved cognition, and experience a better QOL.

As a person increases their activity from 150 to 300 minutes a week, the health benefits become more extensive. For example, a person who does 300 minutes a week has an even lower risk of heart disease or type 2 diabetes than a person who does 150 minutes a week.

Physical Fitness for Adults

Adults who are regularly active at or near the higher end of the key guideline range—300 minutes a week—gain additional health benefits, including further risk reduction for several cancers and prevention of unhealthy weight gain.

The benefits continue to increase with more than 300 minutes a week of moderate-intensity aerobic activity. Research has not identified an upper limit above which additional health benefits cease to occur.

How Many Days a Week and for How Long?
Aerobic physical activity should be spread throughout the week. Research consistently shows that activity performed at least three days a week produces health benefits. Spreading physical activity across at least three days a week may also reduce the risk of injury and prevent excessive fatigue.

All amounts of aerobic activity count toward meeting the key guidelines if they are performed at moderate or vigorous intensity. Episodes of physical activity can be divided throughout the day or week, depending on personal preference.

How Intense Should Your Activity Be?
The key guidelines for adults focus on two levels of intensity—moderate and vigorous. To meet the guidelines, adults can engage in either moderate-intensity or vigorous-intensity aerobic activities, or a combination of both. Vigorous-intensity activities take less time to achieve the same benefit as moderate-intensity activities. A general rule of thumb is that two minutes of moderate-intensity activity is equivalent to one minute of vigorous-intensity activity. For example, 30 minutes of moderate-intensity activity is roughly the same as 15 minutes of vigorous-intensity activity.

The intensity of aerobic activity can be tracked in two ways:
- **Absolute intensity is the amount of energy expended during the activity, without considering a person's cardiorespiratory fitness.** Light-intensity activity expends 1.6–2.9 times the energy used at rest. Moderate-intensity activities expend 3.0–5.9 times

the energy used at rest. Vigorous-intensity activities expend 6.0 or more times the energy used at rest.
- **Relative intensity is the level of effort required to do an activity.** Less fit individuals generally require a higher level of effort than more fit individuals to do the same activity. Relative intensity can be estimated using a scale of 0–10, where sitting is 0 and the highest level of effort possible is 10. Moderate-intensity activity is a 5 or 6, while vigorous-intensity activity begins at 7 or 8.

When using relative intensity, people monitor how physical activity affects their heart rate and breathing. For example, a person doing moderate-intensity aerobic activity can talk but not sing during the activity. A person doing vigorous-intensity activity cannot say more than a few words without pausing for breath.

Table 12.1 lists examples of both moderate- and vigorous-intensity aerobic physical activities, demonstrating the range of exercises that can help improve cardiovascular health.

Table 12.1. Examples of Different Aerobic Physical Activities and Intensities, Based on Absolute Intensity

Moderate-Intensity Activities	Vigorous-Intensity Activities
• Walking briskly (2.5 miles per hour or faster) • Recreational swimming • Bicycling slower than 10 miles per hour on level terrain • Tennis (doubles) • Active forms of yoga • Ballroom or line dancing • General yard work and home repair work • Water aerobics	• Jogging or running • Swimming laps • Tennis (singles) • Vigorous dancing • Bicycling faster than 10 miles per hour • Jumping rope • Heavy yard work • Hiking uphill or with a heavy backpack • High-intensity interval training (HIIT) • Vigorous step aerobics or kickboxing

MUSCLE-STRENGTHENING ACTIVITY

Muscle-strengthening activities provide additional benefits beyond aerobic activity. These benefits include increased bone strength

Physical Fitness for Adults

and muscular fitness. Muscle-strengthening activities can also help maintain muscle mass during weight loss.

Muscle-strengthening activities make muscles work harder than they are accustomed to, thus overloading them. Examples of muscle-strengthening activities include lifting weights, working with resistance bands, doing calisthenics that use body weight for resistance (such as push-ups, pull-ups, and planks), carrying heavy loads, and heavy gardening.

Muscle-strengthening activities count if they involve a moderate or greater level of intensity or effort and work the major muscle groups of the body—the legs, hips, back, chest, abdomen, shoulders, and arms. These activities should be done at least two days a week for all the major muscle groups. The improvement in, or maintenance of, muscle strength is specific to the muscles used during the activity, so a variety of activities is necessary for balanced muscle strength.

No specific amount of time is recommended for muscle strengthening, but exercises should be performed to the point where another repetition would be difficult. When resistance training is used to enhance muscle strength, one set of 8–12 repetitions of each exercise is effective, although two or three sets may be more effective. Increases in the amount of weight or the number of exercise days per week will result in stronger muscles.[1]

Section 12.2 | Preventing Heart Disease in Women through Physical Activity

Heart disease is the leading cause of death for women in the United States, responsible for 310,661 deaths in 2021—about one in every five female deaths. Despite heart disease being the leading cause of death among women in the United States, only about half (56%) of women recognize it as their number one killer. About 1 in 17

---

[1] Office of Disease Prevention and Health Promotion (ODPHP), "Current Guidelines," U.S. Department of Health and Human Services (HHS), August 24, 2021. Available online. URL: https://health.gov/our-work/nutrition-physical-activity/physical-activity-guidelines/current-guidelines. Accessed September 4, 2024.

women aged 20 years and older (5.8%) have coronary artery disease, the most common type of heart disease in the United States.

RECOGNIZING HEART DISEASE SYMPTOMS

Heart disease may sometimes be "silent," not diagnosed until other symptoms or emergencies arise, such as:
- **Heart attack**. Chest pain or discomfort, upper back or neck pain, indigestion, heartburn, nausea or vomiting, extreme fatigue, upper body discomfort, dizziness, and shortness of breath.
- **Arrhythmia**. Fluttering feelings in the chest (palpitations).
- **Heart failure**. Shortness of breath, fatigue, or swelling of the feet, ankles, legs, abdomen, or neck veins.[1]

THE ROLE OF PHYSICAL ACTIVITY IN REDUCING CORONARY HEART DISEASE RISK

Regular moderate- and vigorous-intensity aerobic activity can reduce your risk for coronary heart disease, a condition in which plaque builds up inside the coronary arteries, limiting blood flow to the heart muscle. Over time, plaque buildup can rupture, causing a blood clot that may block blood flow and trigger a heart attack.

Physical activity can help control risk factors for coronary heart disease by:
- lowering blood pressure and triglycerides (a type of fat in the blood)
- raising HDL ("good") cholesterol levels
- reducing the risk of overweight and obesity, when combined with a reduced-calorie diet
- maintaining a healthy weight over time once you have lost weight
- helping your body manage blood sugar and insulin levels, reducing the risk of type 2 diabetes

---

[1] "Lower Your Risk for the Number One Killer of Women," Centers for Disease Control and Prevention (CDC), February 22, 2024. Available online. URL: www.cdc.gov/womens-health/features/heart-disease.html. Accessed September 6, 2024.

- lowering levels of C-reactive protein (CRP), a sign of inflammation and increased heart disease risk
- possibly helping you quit smoking, a major heart disease risk factor

Inactive people are more likely to develop heart disease than those who are physically active. Studies suggest that physical inactivity is a significant risk factor for heart disease, similar to high blood pressure (HBP), high cholesterol, and smoking.

AEROBIC ACTIVITY AND HEART HEALTH FOR HEART DISEASE PATIENTS

Regular aerobic activity helps the heart function better and may reduce the risk of a second heart attack for people with coronary heart disease. However, vigorous aerobic activity may not be safe for all heart disease patients. Consult with your doctor to determine which activities are safe for you and how to incorporate physical activity into your routine.[2]

INCORPORATING CARDIOVASCULAR EXERCISE INTO YOUR ROUTINE

Cardiovascular exercise is crucial to any fitness routine. Aim for at least 30 minutes of moderate-intensity physical activity five or more days a week or 20 minutes of vigorous-intensity physical activity three or more days a week. If 30 minutes a day is too much, studies show that three 10-minute sessions can offer the same benefits as 30 minutes of continuous exercise. No fancy equipment is needed—jumping jacks, running, and dancing are great cardio options that rely only on your body.

REDUCING SITTING TIME FOR BETTER HEALTH

Recent studies reveal that prolonged sitting can harm your health, even if you exercise regularly. Sitting for extended periods has been

---

[2] "Benefits," National Heart, Lung, and Blood Institute (NHLBI), March 24, 2022. Available online. URL: www.nhlbi.nih.gov/health/heart/physical-activity/benefits. Accessed September 6, 2024.

linked to heart attacks, heart disease, and death from cancer. Here are some simple ways to reduce sitting time and improve your health:
- **Break up sitting times.** Get up and move around every 30 minutes.
- **Stand when you can.** Try using a standing desk at work. Many workplaces are offering standing desks to employees.
- **Set reminders to sit less.** At home, get out of your chair during TV commercials. At work, use a smaller coffee cup so you need to make more trips for refills or schedule walking or standing meetings.[3]

Section 12.3 | Physical Activity during Pregnancy and Postpartum

Engaging in physical activity during pregnancy significantly benefits a woman's overall health. Moderate-intensity physical activity among healthy women during pregnancy increases or maintains cardiorespiratory fitness, reduces the risk of excessive weight gain and gestational diabetes, and alleviates symptoms of postpartum depression. By reducing the risk of excessive weight gain during pregnancy, women can also lower the chances of postpartum weight retention, future obesity, and giving birth to infants with high birth weight.

There is strong scientific evidence indicating that moderate-intensity activity poses minimal risks to healthy women during pregnancy. It does not increase the likelihood of low birth weight, preterm delivery, or early pregnancy loss. Some studies suggest that physical activity may reduce the risk of pregnancy complications such as preeclampsia, shorten labor duration, and facilitate postpartum recovery, while also lowering the risk of having a Cesarean section.

---

[3] Smokefree Women, "Get Moving," U.S. Department of Health and Human Services (HHS), September 6, 2018. Available online. URL: https://women.smokefree.gov/live-healthier/care-for-your-body/get-moving. Accessed September 6, 2024.

Physical Fitness for Adults

KEY GUIDELINES FOR WOMEN DURING PREGNANCY AND POSTPARTUM
- During pregnancy and postpartum, women should engage in at least 150 minutes of moderate-intensity aerobic activity per week, which should ideally be distributed throughout the week.
- Women who were habitually involved in vigorous-intensity aerobic activity or were physically active before pregnancy can continue these activities during pregnancy and postpartum.
- Pregnant women should be under the care of a health-care provider who can monitor the progress of the pregnancy and provide guidance on adjusting physical activity.

CLARIFYING THE KEY GUIDELINES
Pregnant women should consult their health-care provider about whether or how to adjust their physical activity during pregnancy and postpartum. Unless a medical condition prevents it, women can begin or continue light- to moderate-intensity aerobic and muscle-strengthening activities, gradually increasing the amount over time.

Women who were engaged in vigorous-intensity or frequent aerobic and muscle-strengthening activity before pregnancy can generally continue being physically active without significantly reducing their activity levels as long as they remain healthy and consult their health-care provider for guidance.

During pregnancy, perceived exertion is a better indicator of intensity than heart rate. On a perceived exertion scale of 0–10, where 0 is resting and 10 is maximal effort, moderate-intensity activity corresponds to an exertion level of five to six. The "talk test" is another way to assess moderate intensity: a woman should be able to converse but not sing while exercising.

Women should avoid exercises that involve lying on their back after the first trimester, as this position may restrict blood flow to the uterus and fetus. Additionally, they should avoid contact or collision sports and activities with a high risk of falling or abdominal trauma, such as soccer, basketball, horseback riding, or downhill skiing.

Fitness and Exercise Sourcebook, Seventh Edition

PHYSICAL ACTIVITY POSTPARTUM

Regular physical activity continues to benefit a woman's health during the postpartum period. Research shows that moderate-intensity physical activity after childbirth improves cardiorespiratory fitness and boosts mood without negatively affecting breast-milk volume, composition, or infant growth. Additionally, physical activity aids women in achieving and maintaining a healthy weight postpartum and, when combined with caloric restriction, supports weight loss.[1]

FREQUENTLY ASKED QUESTIONS

Can You Be Physically Active during Pregnancy and Postpartum?

Yes! Physical activity is beneficial for healthy pregnant and postpartum women. Moderate-intensity physical activity, such as brisk walking, supports heart and lung health during and after pregnancy. It also helps improve mood and supports postpartum weight maintenance and weight loss when combined with healthy eating.

Can You Break Up Your Physical Activity throughout the Week?

Yes! You do not need to do all 150 minutes of aerobic activity at once. Breaking it into smaller sessions, such as 30 minutes of moderate activity five days a week, works just as well. Any amount of moderate or vigorous activity counts toward meeting the weekly guideline.

Is Physical Activity during Pregnancy Risky?

For healthy pregnant women, moderate-intensity aerobic activity, such as brisk walking, poses very low risks. Physical activity does not increase the chances of low birth weight, early delivery, or early pregnancy loss.

---

[1] Office of Disease Prevention and Health Promotion (ODPHP), "Current Guidelines," U.S. Department of Health and Human Services (HHS), August 24, 2021. Available online. URL: https://health.gov/our-work/nutrition-physical-activity/physical-activity-guidelines/current-guidelines. Accessed September 4, 2024.

Physical Fitness for Adults

What Should You Keep in Mind?
Unless a medical reason prevents physical activity, pregnant and postpartum women can begin or continue moderate-intensity aerobic activity.[2]

Section 12.4 | Physical Activity and the Menstrual Cycle

Many women wonder whether it is okay to work out during their period. The answer is simple: yes! In fact, you may find that you can be more physically active and at a greater intensity at certain times of the month than at other times.

DOES MY ENERGY LEVEL CHANGE DURING MY PERIOD?
It might. Some women report low energy levels during their period, while others feel more energetic. Changing hormone levels throughout the menstrual cycle may be the cause.
- **Week 1**. On the first day of your period, estrogen and progesterone levels are at their lowest, but they begin to rise gradually during your period. You may find it easier to be active than in the previous weeks.
- **Week 2**. In the week after your period ends, your energy levels might start to increase. Estrogen levels begin rising quickly in preparation for ovulation.
- **Week 3**. Estrogen levels peak around ovulation, about two weeks before the next period for most women. After ovulation, estrogen levels fall quickly, and progesterone levels rise, which may make you feel more tired or sluggish. This does not mean you should not exercise; being active might boost your mood and give you more energy. Try exercising first thing in the morning before your energy level decreases as the day goes on.

---

[2] "Pregnant and Postpartum Activity: An Overview," Centers for Disease Control and Prevention (CDC), November 28, 2023. Available online. URL: www.cdc.gov/physical-activity-basics/guidelines/healthy-pregnant-or-postpartum-women.html. Accessed September 6, 2024.

- **Week 4**. In the week before your next period, you may feel less energetic as both estrogen and progesterone levels decline (if you are not pregnant). Physical activity may help alleviate premenstrual symptoms (PMS) even if your energy levels are low.

Try keeping a fitness journal to track your menstrual cycle and your energy levels during each workout. After a few months, you should be able to see when you have more or less energy during your cycle.

If you take hormonal birth control, such as the pill, patch, shot, or vaginal ring, your energy levels may still fluctuate with your cycle, but the differences may not be as noticeable.

DOES MY MENSTRUAL CYCLE AFFECT MY ABILITY TO EXERCISE?

No. Researchers have not found any differences in a woman's ability to exercise during different phases of the menstrual cycle. The only significant finding was for endurance events, such as marathons. Women who had already ovulated but had not started their period yet had a harder time exercising in hot and humid weather.

CAN EXERCISE HELP MENSTRUAL CRAMPS?

Maybe. Some women have fewer painful cramps during menstruation if they exercise regularly. Over-the-counter medicines for menstrual cramps or pain work well with very few risks. Regular physical activity, such as walking, also has almost no risks and may help you feel better during your period.

WHAT IF I AM WORKING OUT A LOT AND I DO NOT GET MY PERIOD?

Exercising too much can cause missed menstrual periods or make your periods stop entirely. Irregular or missed periods are more common in athletes and women who train hard regularly. However, if you have not worked out in a long time and suddenly start a vigorous fitness routine, your period could stop or become irregular.

Talk to your doctor or nurse if you have irregular or missed periods. A regular period is a sign of good health. These menstrual issues can lead to more serious health problems, including difficulties getting pregnant and loss of bone density.[1]

Section 12.5 | Managing Weight and Health through Physical Activity

People who are overweight or obese, compared to those with a healthy weight, are at increased risk of many serious diseases and health conditions. These include:
- all-cause mortality (early death)
- high blood pressure (HBP; hypertension)
- high or low LDL cholesterol and high levels of triglycerides (dyslipidemia)
- type 2 diabetes
- coronary heart disease
- stroke
- gallbladder disease
- osteoarthritis
- sleep apnea and breathing problems
- many types of cancers
- lower quality of life (QOL)
- mental illnesses such as clinical depression, anxiety, and other mental disorders
- body pain and difficulty with physical functioning

Body mass index (BMI) is a person's weight in kilograms divided by the square of height in meters. BMI is an inexpensive and easy screening method for the weight category.

---

[1] Office on Women's Health (OWH), "Physical Activity and Your Menstrual Cycle," U.S. Department of Health and Human Services (HHS), February 16, 2021. Available online. URL: www.womenshealth.gov/getting-active/physical-activity-menstrual-cycle#3. Accessed September 6, 2024.

- For people 20 and older, overweight is defined as a BMI between 25 and 30, while obesity is defined as a BMI of 30 or higher.
- For people aged 2–19 years, BMI is defined using age- and sex-specific percentiles from the Centers for Disease Control and Prevention's (CDC) Growth Charts (www.cdc.gov/growthcharts/Extended-BMI-Charts.html). Overweight is defined as a BMI from the 85th percentile to the 95th. Obesity is defined as a BMI at the 95th percentile or higher.[1]

THE BENEFITS OF PHYSICAL ACTIVITY
What Are the Benefits of Physical Activity?

Experts recommend that you should move more and sit less throughout the day. Even a small amount of physical activity can provide health benefits. Being physically active can help you feel better immediately by:
- boosting your mood
- sharpening your focus
- reducing your stress
- improving your sleep

Regular physical activity can lead to even more health benefits over time, such as:
- helping prevent heart disease and stroke
- controlling your blood pressure
- lowering your risk of diseases such as type 2 diabetes and some cancers

What Types of Physical Activity Do I Need?

Experts recommend two types of physical activities: aerobic and muscle-strengthening activities.

---

[1] "How Overweight and Obesity Impacts Your Health," Centers for Disease Control and Prevention (CDC), January 4, 2024. Available online. URL: www.cdc.gov/healthy-weight-growth/food-activity/overweight-obesity-impacts-health.html. Accessed September 6, 2024.

Physical Fitness for Adults

AEROBIC ACTIVITY
Also known as "endurance" or "cardio activities," these use large muscle groups (chest, legs, and back) to increase your heart rate and breathing. Aerobic activities can be moderate or vigorous. Use the "talk test" to gauge intensity: if you can talk but not sing, it is moderate-intensity; if you can only say a few words before needing a breath, it is vigorous. Start with moderate-intensity and gradually work up to vigorous-intensity to avoid injuries.

Examples include:
- brisk walking or jogging
- bicycling
- swimming
- dancing
- playing basketball or soccer
- hiking

Regular aerobic activity can help you manage your weight, prevent heart disease and stroke, lower the risk of type 2 diabetes and some cancers, and maintain strong bones.

MUSCLE-STRENGTHENING ACTIVITY
Strength training, or resistance training, works your muscles by making you push or pull against resistance, such as weights, exercise bands, or your own body weight.

Examples include:
- lifting weights (e.g., using cans of food or water containers)
- doing push-ups, pull-ups, or planks
- working with resistance bands
- engaging in heavy gardening (digging, lifting, carrying)
- climbing stairs or hills

Regular muscle-strengthening activities can increase bone strength, prevent bone loss, maintain muscle mass, and engage major muscle groups such as the chest, back, abdominals, legs, and arms.

BEING GOOD TO YOURSELF

Many people experience stress in their daily lives, which can lead to overeating, fatigue, and a lack of motivation to be active. Healthy eating and regular physical activity can help manage stress.

Try these additional strategies to relieve stress and stay healthy:
- Get adequate sleep.
- Try a new hobby or activity that interests you.
- Surround yourself with people whose company you enjoy.
- Explore apps that offer tips on stress management and help monitor stress triggers.

A balanced eating plan, regular physical activity, stress relief, adequate sleep, and other positive behaviors can help you maintain good health for life.[2]

---

[2] "Health Tips for Adults," National Institute of Diabetes and Digestive and Kidney Diseases (NIDDK), September 2020. Available online. URL: www.niddk.nih.gov/health-information/weight-management/healthy-eating-physical-activity-for-life/health-tips-for-adults?dkrd=/health-information/weight-management/health-tips-adults#activity. Accessed September 6, 2024.

Chapter 13 | Physical Fitness for Older Adults

Chapter Contents
Section 13.1—Promoting Physical Activity for Healthy Aging ...107
Section 13.2—Exercise and Well-Being for Older Adults.........111
Section 13.3—Ensuring Safety in Physical Activity for Older Adults..115
Section 13.4—Safety Tips for Exercising Outdoors for Older Adults..119
Section 13.5—The Heart Benefits of Light Physical Activity for Older Women 121

Section 13.1 | **Promoting Physical Activity for Healthy Aging**

BENEFITS OF REGULAR PHYSICAL ACTIVITY

The benefits of regular physical activity occur throughout life and are essential for healthy aging. Adults aged 65 years and older gain substantial health benefits from regular physical activity. However, it is never too late to start being physically active. Being physically active makes it easier to perform activities of daily living, including eating, bathing, toileting, dressing, getting into or out of a bed or chair, and moving around the house or neighborhood. Physically active older adults are less likely to experience falls, and if they do fall, they are less likely to be seriously injured. Physical activity can also preserve physical function and mobility, which may help maintain independence longer and delay the onset of major disability. Research shows that physical activity can improve physical function in adults of any age, including those with overweight or obesity, and even those who are frail. Promoting physical activity and reducing sedentary behavior for older adults is especially important because this population is the least physically active of any age group, and most older adults spend a significant proportion of their day being sedentary.

MANAGING CHRONIC CONDITIONS AND ENHANCING QUALITY OF LIFE

Older adults are a varied group. Most, but not all, have one or more chronic conditions, such as type 2 diabetes, cardiovascular disease, osteoarthritis, or cancer, and these conditions vary in type and severity. Nevertheless, being physically active has significant benefits for all older adults. Physical activity is key to preventing and managing chronic disease. Other benefits include a lower risk of dementia, better-perceived quality of life (QOL), and reduced symptoms of anxiety and depression. Additionally, doing physical activity with others can provide opportunities for social engagement and interaction. All older adults experience a loss of physical fitness and function with age, but some experience this more than others. This diversity means that some older adults can run several miles, while others struggle to walk a few blocks.

KEY GUIDELINES FOR OLDER ADULTS

- Move more and sit less throughout the day. Some physical activity is better than none. Adults who sit less and engage in any amount of moderate-to-vigorous physical activity gain some health benefits.
- For substantial health benefits, adults should do at least 150 minutes (2 hours and 30 minutes) to 300 minutes (5 hours) a week of moderate-intensity aerobic physical activity, or 75 minutes (1 hour and 15 minutes) to 150 minutes (2 hours and 30 minutes) a week of vigorous-intensity aerobic physical activity, or an equivalent combination of moderate- and vigorous-intensity aerobic activity. Preferably, aerobic activity should be spread throughout the week. Additional health benefits are gained by engaging in physical activity beyond the equivalent of 300 minutes (5 hours) of moderate-intensity physical activity a week.
- Adults should also do muscle-strengthening activities of moderate or greater intensity that involve all major muscle groups on two or more days a week, as these activities provide additional health benefits.
- Older adults should engage in multicomponent physical activity that includes balance training, aerobic exercise, and muscle-strengthening activities as part of their weekly routine.
- Older adults should determine their level of effort for physical activity relative to their level of fitness. Older adults with chronic conditions should understand whether and how their conditions affect their ability to do regular physical activity safely.
- When older adults cannot do 150 minutes of moderate-intensity aerobic activity a week because of chronic conditions, they should be as physically active as their abilities and conditions allow.

Physical Fitness for Older Adults

EXAMPLES OF PHYSICAL ACTIVITIES FOR OLDER ADULTS
Aerobic Activities
- walking or hiking
- dancing
- swimming
- water aerobics
- jogging or running
- aerobic exercise classes
- some forms of yoga
- bicycle riding (stationary or outdoors)
- some yard work, such as raking and pushing a lawn mower
- sports such as tennis or basketball
- walking as part of the golf

Muscle-Strengthening Activities
- strengthening exercises using exercise bands, weight machines, or hand-held weights
- body-weight exercises (push-ups, pull-ups, planks, squats, lunges)
- digging, lifting, and carrying as part of gardening
- carrying groceries
- some yoga postures
- some forms of tai chi

WHAT IS MULTICOMPONENT PHYSICAL ACTIVITY?
For older adults, multicomponent physical activity is important to improve physical function and decrease the risk of falls or injury from a fall. These activities can be done at home or in a structured group setting. Many studied interventions combine all types of exercise (aerobic, muscle strengthening, and balance) into one session, and this has been shown to be effective.

Examples of a multicomponent physical activity program could include:
- walking (aerobic activity)
- lifting weights (muscle strengthening)

- incorporating balance exercises by walking backwards or sideways, or by standing on one foot while doing an upper-body muscle-strengthening activity, such as bicep curls
- ballroom dancing, which combines aerobic and balance components

ENCOURAGING AN ACTIVE LIFESTYLE

Older adults have many options for living an active lifestyle that meets the key guidelines. Many factors influence decisions to be active, such as personal goals, current physical activity habits, and health and safety considerations. In all cases, older adults should try to move more and sit less each day. When working toward meeting the key guidelines, older adults are encouraged to do a variety of activities. This approach can make physical activity more enjoyable and may reduce the risk of overuse injury.

Healthy older adults who plan gradual increases in their weekly amounts of physical activity generally do not need to consult a health-care professional before becoming physically active. However, health-care professionals and physical activity specialists can help people attain and maintain regular physical activity by providing advice on appropriate types of activities and ways to progress at a safe and steady pace.

Older adults with chronic conditions should talk with their health-care professional to determine whether their conditions limit, in any way, their ability to do regular physical activity. Such a conversation can also help individuals learn about appropriate types and amounts of physical activity.[1]

---

[1] Office of Disease Prevention and Health Promotion (ODPHP), "Physical Activity Guidelines for Americans, 2nd Edition," U.S. Department of Health and Human Services (HHS), 2018. Available online. URL: https://health.gov/paguidelines/second-edition/pdf/Physical_Activity_Guidelines_2nd_edition.pdf#page=66. Accessed September 6, 2024.

Physical Fitness for Older Adults

Section 13.2 | Exercise and Well-Being for Older Adults

WHY IS PHYSICAL ACTIVITY SO IMPORTANT?

Eating a nutritious diet and maintaining a healthy weight are only part of a healthy lifestyle. Almost anyone at any age can exercise safely and gain meaningful benefits.

Research shows that regular physical activity, including exercise, is important to the physical, emotional, and mental health of almost everyone. As you age, being physically active can help you stay strong and fit, allowing you to continue doing the things you enjoy and maintain your independence.

In fact, studies show that "taking it easy" is risky. Often, inactivity is more to blame than age when older adults lose the ability to do things on their own. Regular physical activity over long periods can produce lasting health benefits. That is why health experts say that older adults should remain regularly active throughout each week to maintain optimal health.

EMOTIONAL AND COGNITIVE BENEFITS OF PHYSICAL ACTIVITY

Physical activities—such as walking, biking, dancing, yoga, or tai chi—can improve your mood and overall emotional well-being, help reduce feelings of depression and stress, increase your energy levels, improve your sleep, and empower you to feel more in control. Additionally, exercise and physical activity may improve or help maintain some aspects of cognitive function, such as your ability to shift quickly between tasks, focus your attention on a new activity, or plan an outing with friends or family members.

PREVENTING AND MANAGING CHRONIC CONDITIONS THROUGH EXERCISE

Moreover, regular exercise and physical activity can reduce the risk of developing some diseases and disabilities associated with aging. In some cases, exercise can help manage chronic conditions. For example, studies show that people with heart disease, arthritis, and diabetes benefit from regular exercise. Exercise also helps people with high blood pressure (HBP), balance problems, and difficulty walking.

PRACTICAL WAYS TO STAY ACTIVE

Research shows the benefits of physical activity extend beyond physical well-being. Exercise and physical activity support emotional and mental health.

For example, you can be active in short spurts throughout the day, or you can set aside specific times on certain days of the week to exercise. Many physical activities—such as brisk walking, raking leaves, or taking the stairs whenever you can—are free or low-cost and do not require special equipment. You could also try a workout video on YouTube or another online service at home. Alternatively, try contacting your local fitness center, senior center, or parks and recreation department about facilities and programs in your area, which may offer senior discounts. Staying safe while you exercise is important, whether you are starting a new activity or have been active for a long time.

HOW MUCH ACTIVITY DO OLDER ADULTS NEED?

Today, we know a lot more about older adults and their need to exercise. Regardless of health and physical abilities, older adults can benefit from staying physically active. Even if you have difficulty standing or walking, you can still exercise and reap the benefits. In fact, in most cases, you have more to lose by not doing anything! According to the *Physical Activity Guidelines for Americans*, you should do at least 150 minutes (2½ hours) a week of moderate-intensity aerobic activity, such as brisk walking or fast dancing. Being active at least three days a week is ideal, but doing anything is better than doing nothing at all. You should also do muscle-strengthening activities, such as lifting weights or doing push-ups, at least two days a week. The *Physical Activity Guidelines for Americans* recommends that, as part of your weekly physical activity, you include multicomponent activities that incorporate balance training, as well as aerobic and muscle-strengthening exercises. If you prefer vigorous-intensity aerobic activity (such as running), aim for at least 75 minutes a week.

FIT PHYSICAL ACTIVITY INTO YOUR EVERYDAY LIFE

There are many ways to fit a little physical activity into your day. To get the most out of your efforts, physical activity needs to become a regular part of your life.

Here are some ideas to help:

Make It a Priority

Being active is one of the most important things you can do each day to maintain and improve your health.

Among many other benefits, physical activity can:
- make your muscles stronger
- increase your heart rate
- improve your balance
- stretch your muscles

Make It Easy

You are more likely to exercise if it is a convenient part of your day.
- Walk every aisle of the grocery store when you go shopping.
- Try being active first thing in the morning before you get too busy.
- Combine physical activity with a task that is already part of your day, such as walking the dog or doing household chores.
- Join a gym or local senior center that is close to your home and easy to access.
- Go for a hike in a park or walk up and down stairs (such as one up and two down).
- Make your own weights with water bottles or other household items.

Make It Social
Many people agree that an "exercise buddy" helps keep them motivated and provides emotional support.
- Take a walk during lunch with co-workers.
- Try a dance class—salsa, tango, or square dancing—it is up to you.
- Use family gatherings as a time to play team sports or do outdoor activities.
- Try two-person activities, such as playing tennis.
- If group activities appeal to you, try a sport such as pickleball or join an exercise class or local recreational sports league.
- Set regular meetups to exercise as a group for accountability and camaraderie.
- Participate in a community-sponsored cleanup or fun run/walk.
- Walk or roll with friends or family at the mall or around your neighborhood.
- Start a walking club with friends or organize an exercise class at your local library.

Make It Fun
Do activities you enjoy to make exercise more fun. If you love the outdoors, try biking or hiking, or listen to music while you garden or wash the car.

BENEFITS OF EXERCISE AND PHYSICAL ACTIVITY
Exercise and physical activity benefit every area of your life. Staying active can help you:
- maintain and improve your strength, so you can remain as independent as possible
- have more energy to do the things you want to do and reduce fatigue
- improve your balance, lower your risk of falls, and reduce injuries from falls
- manage and prevent some diseases, such as arthritis, heart disease, stroke, type 2 diabetes, osteoporosis,

Physical Fitness for Older Adults

and certain types of cancer, including breast and colon cancer
- boost your mood and reduce feelings of depression
- sleep better at night
- reduce stress and anxiety
- lose weight or reduce weight gain when combined with a reduced calorie intake
- control your blood pressure
- possibly improve or maintain some aspects of cognitive function, such as your ability to shift quickly between tasks or plan an activity[1]

Section 13.3 | Ensuring Safety in Physical Activity for Older Adults

PHYSICAL ACTIVITY FOR OLDER ADULTS

People can begin or restart physical activity at any age, and older adults have many options for leading an active lifestyle that aligns with key guidelines. Participating in a structured exercise class, gardening, walking to the bus for an appointment, and playing with grandchildren are all ways to move more throughout the day. Healthy older adults who plan gradual increases in their weekly physical activity generally do not need to consult a clinician before becoming active. However, clinicians and exercise professionals can support individuals in attaining and maintaining regular physical activity by advising on appropriate activities and ways to progress safely and steadily. Older adults with chronic conditions should be under the care of a health-care provider and can consult their clinician to determine whether their conditions limit their ability to engage in regular physical activity.

In general, people who engage in physical activity can protect themselves by using appropriate gear and sports equipment,

---

[1] National Institute on Aging (NIA), "Get Fit for Life," National Institutes of Health (NIH), January 1, 2024. Available online. URL: https://order.nia.nih.gov/sites/default/files/2024-05/get-fit-life-book.pdf. Accessed September 6, 2024.

choosing safe environments, following rules and policies, and making sensible decisions about when, where, and how to be active. Additionally, to reduce the risk of injuries and other adverse events, older adults can choose physical activities that are suitable for their current fitness level and health goals. Starting with lower-intensity activities and gradually increasing the frequency, intensity, and duration of activities can help reduce the risk of injury.

BARRIERS TO PHYSICAL ACTIVITY

Several barriers can affect an individual's perceived or actual ability to engage in physical activity. For older adults, these barriers often relate to capabilities (i.e., individual attributes), opportunities (i.e., external factors), or motivation (i.e., personal attitudes and beliefs). Understanding these barriers is essential to delivering effective and equitable interventions.

Barriers to physical activity vary among individuals and are influenced by socioeconomic, cultural, environmental, and community factors. For example, some people may not be aware of or have access to safe places to be active, while others may live in communities that are not conducive to physical activity or have physical or cognitive limitations. Additionally, access to specialized facilities or equipment—especially for muscle-strengthening activities—can be costly. Older adults may face unique concerns, such as the fear of falling, safety issues, or challenges related to chronic health conditions, mobility, and pain. Neighborhood characteristics, such as poor-quality sidewalks or insufficient lighting, can reduce perceived or actual safety. Other common barriers include a lack of time, unfavorable weather, and lack of enjoyment.

Societal expectations about the types of physical activity that older adults can participate in may contribute to a lack of social support. In addition to age, intersecting social identities such as ability, race, and gender or sexual identity may interact with environments to influence feelings of safety, belonging, and inclusion. Not feeling safe or comfortable in public spaces may reduce opportunities for physical activity. Racism—both interpersonal and structural—negatively affects the mental and physical health of millions, preventing them from achieving their highest level of health, which, in turn, affects the health of the nation.

Getting and staying active can be particularly challenging as people age, and the barriers older adults face cannot be addressed with a single strategy or in one setting. The strategies outlined in this report can be combined and tailored to different community contexts and settings. By directly engaging with communities experiencing inequities and continuing to explore barriers, individuals and organizations from various sectors can use these strategies to help older adults overcome obstacles to physical activity and become more active.

EQUITY AND PHYSICAL ACTIVITY

Not everyone has equal access to safe spaces for physical activity. Different racial and ethnic groups experience unequal rates of physical activity. These disparities exist partly because many people live in neighborhoods lacking safe spaces or other social and environmental supports for physical activity. Even in areas with safe spaces, some people may be excluded. For instance, recreation areas may not be designed for older adults or people with disabilities, contributing to disparities in physical activity. Some older adults with low incomes or those living in rural areas may not have access to broadband, restricting their ability to participate in virtual physical activity programs or online exercise communities that provide opportunities for social connection. Severe weather events and temperature extremes associated with climate change may disproportionately affect certain populations or geographic areas. People also have multiple social identities, including age, ability status, race, gender, income level, and religious affiliation. In addition to physical barriers, these intersecting identities and historical contexts may interact with environments to influence feelings of safety, belonging, and inclusion. If people do not see others who resemble them in public spaces (i.e., a lack of representation), they may not feel welcome. Feeling unsafe or uncomfortable in public spaces due to ageism, racism, sexism, or ableism may reduce opportunities for physical activity. Engaging with people, groups, and organizations most affected by inequities can improve understanding of these experiences.

COMMUNITY DESIGN

One effective strategy for increasing physical activity among older adults is making communities more walkable through thoughtful community design. Researchers have found that people who live in walkable neighborhoods are more active than those who do not. Walkable neighborhoods make it safer and easier for community members to walk, bike, or use wheelchairs for recreation, fitness, or transportation.

Community design elements that improve walkability include:
- availability of and access to everyday destinations
- sidewalk connectivity, quality, and networks
- social, aesthetic, and functional components

Walkable neighborhoods provide easy access to a mix of destinations, such as affordable housing options, cultural centers, food outlets, health-care institutions, parks, trails, recreational facilities, and retailers. These neighborhoods also feature connected networks of "activity-friendly routes," such as safe, accessible, high-quality sidewalks, curbs, intersections, multi-use trails, safe bicycle infrastructure, and convenient public transit. For instance, intersections may include clearly marked crosswalks, curb cuts that eliminate the need to step up onto a sidewalk from the road, and walk signals with audio and visual prompts that allow sufficient crossing time. These features help people—especially those who use mobility devices or have mobility impairments—safely cross the street. Wide sidewalks with adequate lighting and free of hazards such as cracks or overgrowth also improve walkability, creating safer, smoother paths for older adults using wheelchairs and other assistive devices. Walkable communities can include social, aesthetic, and functional features that contribute to perceptions of safety and inclusion, such as benches, public art, gathering spaces, shade, landscaping, access to bathrooms, and safe, free drinking water.

With a combination of inclusive community design and tailored strategies that engage those most affected by inequities, it is possible to create safe, supportive environments that encourage physical activity for all older adults, helping them lead healthier, more active lives.[1]

Section 13.4 | Safety Tips for Exercising Outdoors for Older Adults

Staying active is important for health, and exercising outdoors can be a great way to get moving. However, it is crucial to ensure safety while doing so. Here are some tips to help older adults exercise safely outdoors.

GENERAL SAFETY TIPS
Think Ahead about Safety
- Carry your identification (ID) with emergency contact information and bring a small amount of cash and a cell phone, especially if walking alone.
- Stay alert by avoiding phone conversations and keeping the volume low on headphones.
- Let others know where you are going and when you plan to return.
- Stick to well-lit places with other people around.

Be Seen to Be Safe
- Wear light or brightly colored clothing during the day.
- Wear reflective material on your clothing and carry a flashlight at night.
- Put lights on the front and back of your bike.
- Wear sturdy, appropriate shoes for your activity that provide proper footing.

---

[1] Office of Disease Prevention and Health Promotion (ODPHP), "Physical Activity Guidelines for Americans Midcourse Report: Implementation Strategies for Older Adults," U.S. Department of Health and Human Services (HHS), August 2023. Available online. URL: https://health.gov/sites/default/files/2023-08/PAG_MidcourseReport_508c_08-10.pdf. Accessed September 6, 2024.

TIPS FOR WALKING SAFELY IN RURAL AREAS
- Walk during daylight hours whenever possible.
- Choose routes that are well-used, well-lit, and safe, with places to sit if you need to rest.
- Stay alert at all times. If listening to music, keep the volume low to hear warnings from others.
- Always walk facing oncoming traffic.
- Use sidewalks or paths whenever possible, and watch out for uneven surfaces.
- Look for a smooth, stable surface alongside the road.

TIPS FOR WALKING SAFELY IN URBAN AREAS
- If the road has guardrails, walk on a smooth, flat surface behind the barrier. Stay as far from traffic as possible on a paved shoulder.
- Watch for bridges and narrow shoulders.
- Cross at crosswalks or intersections and pay attention to traffic signals. Cross only when you have the pedestrian crossing signal.
- Make eye contact with drivers before crossing and ensure you have plenty of time to get across.
- Look left, right, and left again before crossing multiple lanes. Do not assume all drivers will stop for you.
- Check out city parks for walking or jogging trails away from traffic.

BICYCLE SAFETY FOR OLDER ADULTS
Riding a bicycle is a fun way to exercise and can be used for commuting or errands. To stay safe while cycling:
- Wear a helmet that fits properly.
- Use lights and reflectors to increase visibility.
- Follow traffic rules, signal turns, and ride in bike lanes when available.
- Stay alert for pedestrians, other cyclists, and vehicles.

Physical Fitness for Older Adults

TIPS FOR EXERCISING IN HOT WEATHER
- Check the weather forecast. If it is very hot or humid, consider exercising indoors or walking in an air-conditioned space like a shopping mall.
- Drink plenty of water and fruit juices, avoiding caffeine and alcohol.
- Wear light-colored, loose-fitting clothes made from natural fabrics.
- Dress in layers, so you can remove clothing as your body warms up.
- Be aware of signs of heat-related illnesses, such as heat stroke or heat exhaustion, and seek medical help if necessary.

TIPS FOR EXERCISING IN COLD WEATHER
- Check the weather forecast. If it is very cold or windy, exercise indoors or plan to go out at a later time.
- Watch out for snow and icy sidewalks to avoid slipping.
- Warm up your muscles before going out, such as by walking or light arm pumping.
- Dress in several layers of loose clothing to trap warm air. Avoid tight clothing, which can restrict blood flow and lead to heat loss.
- Wear a waterproof coat or jacket if it is snowy or rainy, and use a hat, scarf, and gloves to protect against the cold.[1]

Section 13.5 | The Heart Benefits of Light Physical Activity for Older Women

HOW LIGHT ACTIVITY CAN LOWER CARDIOVASCULAR RISKS
Light physical activity, such as gardening, strolling through a park, and folding clothes, might be enough to significantly lower the

---

[1] National Institute on Aging (NIA), "Safety Tips for Exercising Outdoors for Older Adults," National Institutes of Health (NIH), April 2, 2020. Available online. URL: www.nia.nih.gov/health/exercise-and-physical-activity/safety-tips-exercising-outdoors-older-adults. Accessed September 6, 2024.

risk of cardiovascular disease among women aged 63 and older, a recent study found. This type of activity, researchers said, appears to reduce the risk of cardiovascular events such as stroke or heart failure by up to 22 percent and the risk of heart attack or coronary death by as much as 42 percent.

The results of the study, funded by the National Heart, Lung, and Blood Institute (NHLBI), part of the National Institutes of Health, were published in the journal *JAMA Network Open*.

"When we tell people to move with heart, we mean it, and the supporting evidence keeps growing," said David Goff, MD, PhD, director of the Division of Cardiovascular Sciences at NHLBI. "This study suggests that for older women, any and all movement counts towards better cardiovascular health," Goff added that the findings align with the federal government's most recent physical activity guidelines, which encourage replacing sedentary behavior with light physical activity whenever possible.

IMPORTANCE OF LIGHT PHYSICAL ACTIVITY

Heart disease is the leading cause of death among American women, with nearly 68 percent of those aged 60–79 affected. Older adults are also heavily affected, with more than half of the estimated 85.6 million adults with at least one type of cardiovascular disease being 60 or older.

The study involved a diverse group of 5,861 women enrolled between 2012 and 2014, none of whom had a history of myocardial infarction or stroke. These women were part of the NHLBI-funded Objective Physical Activity and Cardiovascular Health (OPACH), a sub-cohort of the Women's Health Initiative.

Participants wore hip-mounted accelerometers, similar to fitness trackers, that measured their movement 24 hours a day for seven consecutive days. The accelerometers were calibrated by age to distinguish between light and moderate-to-vigorous physical activity. The researchers then followed the participants for almost five years, tracking cardiovascular disease events such as heart attacks and strokes.

"To our knowledge, this is the first study to investigate light physical activity measured by accelerometer in relation to fatal and

Physical Fitness for Older Adults

non-fatal coronary heart disease in older women," said LaCroix, who led the OPACH study.

Previous studies largely relied on self-reporting questionnaires, which may not capture light physical activities such as folding clothes or walking to the mailbox. "There was no correlation between the amount of self-reported light physical activity and the amount measured with accelerometers," LaCroix noted. "Without accurate reporting, we risk discounting low-intensity activities associated with important heart health benefits."

Researchers need to conduct large randomized trials to determine if specific interventions could increase light physical activity in older women and what effect this would have on cardiovascular disease rates. However, the OPACH authors encourage older women to increase their light physical activity immediately.[1]

---

[1] News and Events, "Light Physical Activity Linked to Lower Risk of Heart Disease in Older Women," National Institutes of Health (NIH), March 15, 2019. Available online. URL: www.nih.gov/news-events/news-releases/light-physical-activity-linked-lower-risk-heart-disease-older-women. Accessed September 6, 2024.

Part 3 | **Start Moving**

Chapter 14 | **Building an Active Lifestyle**

Chapter Contents
Section 14.1—Incorporating Physical Activity into
 Daily Life 129
Section 14.2—Getting Active and Overcoming Physical
 Activity Roadblocks 133
Section 14.3—Making Exercise a Shared Enjoyment 136

Section 14.1 | Incorporating Physical Activity into Daily Life

ADDING PHYSICAL ACTIVITY TO DAILY LIFE

There are many ways adults can incorporate physical activity into their lives. Any aerobic activity counts as long as it is done at a moderate or vigorous intensity. Any amount of physical activity provides health benefits. Physical activity supports both physical and mental health. The benefits make it one of the most important things you can do for your overall well-being.

According to the *Physical Activity Guidelines for Americans*, adults need 150 minutes of moderate-intensity physical activity and two days of muscle-strengthening activities each week. The 150 minutes can be broken up. For example, you could be physically active for 30 minutes a day, five days a week. Some physical activity is better than none. You might be surprised by how many ways there are to get the recommended amount of physical activity each week.

STICK WITH IT

To ensure consistency, choose physical activities that you enjoy and that match your abilities. If you are unsure where to start, here are some examples of weekly physical activity schedules for adults that meet the recommended levels of aerobic and muscle-strengthening activities.

Example 1. Figure 14.1 illustrates the recommended weekly combination of 150 minutes of moderate-intensity aerobic activity along with two days of muscle-strengthening exercises.

Example 2. Figure 14.2 demonstrates the recommended weekly combination of 75 minutes of vigorous-intensity aerobic activity along with two days of muscle-strengthening exercises.

Example 3. Figure 14.3 outlines a balanced approach to physical fitness, combining the equivalent of 150 minutes of moderate-intensity aerobic activity with two days of muscle-strengthening exercises per week.

Fitness and Exercise Sourcebook, Seventh Edition

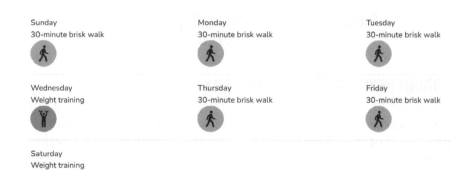

Figure 14.1. Moderate-Intensity Activity and Muscle-Strengthening Activity
Centers for Disease Control and Prevention (CDC)

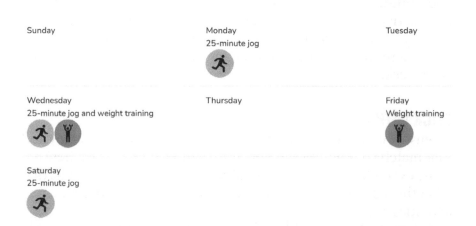

Figure 14.2. Vigorous-Intensity Activity and Muscle-Strengthening Activity
Centers for Disease Control and Prevention (CDC)

WHEN TO CHECK WITH YOUR DOCTOR

Moderate physical activity is safe for most people. However, if you have a chronic health condition, be sure to consult your doctor about the types and amounts of physical activity that are right for you. Examples of chronic conditions include heart disease, arthritis, and diabetes.

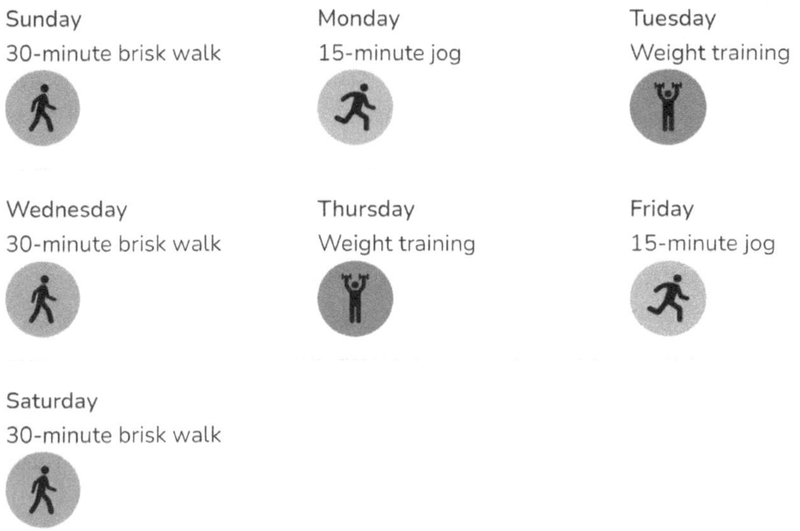

Building an Active Lifestyle

Sunday
30-minute brisk walk

Monday
15-minute jog

Tuesday
Weight training

Wednesday
30-minute brisk walk

Thursday
Weight training

Friday
15-minute jog

Saturday
30-minute brisk walk

Figure 14.3. Mix of Aerobic and Muscle-Strengthening Activity
Centers for Disease Control and Prevention (CDC)

It is also advisable to talk to your doctor before starting vigorous-intensity physical activity if you have been inactive, have a disability, or are overweight.[1]

HOW YOUR NEIGHBORHOOD AFFECTS PHYSICAL ACTIVITY

Studies have found that your neighborhood can influence your level of activity. Researchers have investigated what makes a neighborhood "walkable."

"We found that things like having destinations close to where you live certainly encourage more walking," says Dr. Brian Saelens of the University of Washington and Seattle Children's Research Institute. For example, people are more likely to walk to a nearby store.

---

[1] "Adding Physical Activity as an Adult," Centers for Disease Control and Prevention (CDC), January 8, 2024. Available online. URL: www.cdc.gov/physical-activity-basics/adding-adults. Accessed September 7, 2024.

Saelens' team studies how the environment influences physical activity and eating habits. "Walkable neighborhoods also have more connected street networks," he says, "so it's easy to get from point A to point B without taking a long route around." His research also suggests that children are more physically active when they live near parks and playgrounds.

FINDING MOTIVATION AND STRATEGIES FOR STAYING ACTIVE

Knowing you should be more active and actually doing it are two different things. Studies have found that effective approaches vary from person to person.

"One solution that works for one person may not work for others," notes Dr. Chen. Some people find it motivating to use wearable devices or phone apps to track progress. Others may benefit from joining a group that engages in physical activity together.

Making physical activity social can make it more enjoyable and less like a chore. Try to find someone you enjoy being active with. This can be especially important for children, who are more likely to be active when with others.

Parents play a key role in keeping their children active. "Parents need to model being active and provide opportunities for activity," Saelens says. Invite your child to take a walk with you. Even if they do not join, you are modeling the behavior.

If low energy is keeping you from being active, schedule exercise for the time of day when you have the most energy. Remind yourself that physical activity usually increases energy levels. So, find what works for you. It could be riding bikes with a friend, dancing, or taking a midday stroll.

"Any activity is better than no activity," says Dr. Jakicic. "Do not look for the magic bullet. Look for what fits into your lifestyle, find what works for you, and try to build on that every day."

Here are some tips for making your day more active:
- Set specific goals for your physical activity. This increases the likelihood that you will meet them.
- Take the stairs instead of the elevator.
- Park your car at the far end of the street or parking lot.

Building an Active Lifestyle

- Make your screen time more active. Set up your space so you can walk on a treadmill while watching TV or stand when using the computer.
- Try an online exercise class to stay active from home.
- Set an alarm to go off every hour as a reminder to move around for a minute or two.
- Keep small weights in your office or around your home for arm exercises.
- Take a walk during your lunch breaks or have "walking meetings" with colleagues at work.[2]

Section 14.2 | Getting Active and Overcoming Physical Activity Roadblocks

WHY SHOULD YOU BE PHYSICALLY ACTIVE?

Physical activity is an important step you can take to improve your health and quality of life (QOL). Regular physical activity may help prevent or delay many health problems. Being active can help you look and feel better, both now and in the future.

So what is stopping you? Perhaps you think physical activity is boring, joining a gym is costly, or fitting one more thing into your busy day seems impossible. This information may help you identify and overcome your roadblocks to physical activity!

HOW CAN YOU OVERCOME PHYSICAL ACTIVITY ROADBLOCKS?

Starting a physical activity program and sticking with it may be easier than you think. You can overcome these common roadblocks to physical activity.

---

[2] *NIH News in Health*, "Step It Up!" National Institutes of Health (NIH), July 2021. Available online. URL: https://newsinhealth.nih.gov/2021/07/step-it-up. Accessed September 7, 2024.

Fitness and Exercise Sourcebook, Seventh Edition

You Do Not Have Time

Are work, family, and other demands making it hard to be active? Try the tips below to add physical activity to your daily routine. Remember, every bit counts.
- **Do 10 minutes of physical activity at a time**. Spread bursts of activity throughout your day.
- **Add a 15-minute walk or activity during your lunch break or after dinner that you will stick with.**
- **Make activity part of your daily routine**. If it is safe and you have time, walk a flight of stairs or, instead of driving, walk or bike with your child to school. If you have a physical disability, you can use aids to incorporate activity into your daily routine.

You Are Not That Motivated or Interested

Do you find it hard to get moving? Does working out seem like a chore? Here are some ideas to keep you motivated:
- **Switch it up**. Try a new activity, such as dancing or water aerobics, to discover what you enjoy most.
- **Make it social**. Involve your family and friends. Physical activity is good for them, too. Plan fun activities that allow you to spend quality time together and stay on track.
- **Meet a friend for workouts or train together for a charity event.**
- **Join a class or sports league where people count on you to show up.**
- **No matter what age your kids are, find an activity you can do together**. Dance to music or play sports such as basketball or tennis, even in a wheelchair if needed.
- **Seek support**. Who will inspire you to get moving and help you reach your goals?
- **Make a list of people—your partner, siblings, parents, kids, or friends—who can support your efforts to be physically active**. Give them ideas on how they can help, such as praising your efforts, watching your kids, or working out with you.

Building an Active Lifestyle

It Is Too Cold, Hot, or Rainy
You can reach your fitness goals in any weather.
- **Wear the right gear.** A rain jacket, sun hat and sunscreen, or winter clothes will protect you and help you stick to your plans.
- **Find a place to stay active indoors.** Download an app to your phone or other device to stay active at home, or take an indoor class when the weather is bad. Your local community center or place of worship may offer low-cost options.

You Are Afraid It Will Cost Too Much
Getting physical activity does not have to be expensive.
- **Check out your local recreation (rec) or community center.** These centers may cost less than other gyms or fitness centers. Find one that lets you pay only for the months or classes you want, rather than the whole year. If you have a physical disability, ask if the center offers activities that suit your abilities.
- **Choose physical activities that do not require special gear or advanced skills.** Turn on some music and host a dance party with friends and family.

BREAKING THROUGH BARRIERS
What are the top three things keeping you from being more active? Use your phone, calendar, or computer to make a list of barriers that come to mind and how you can overcome them. For example:
- **Barrier**: I do not have anyone to watch my kids.
- **Solution**: Be active with your child. You can take walks together or play games such as "catch" or basketball. You can also try seated activities such as wheelchair volleyball. Lifting or carrying a baby not only works your muscles but also helps you bond with your child. Some rec centers offer "baby and me" classes. Another option is to find child care. Ask whether your rec center has child care, or find a trusted friend or family

Fitness and Exercise Sourcebook, Seventh Edition

member who is willing to watch your child while you exercise. Some people take turns watching each other's children.

Set specific goals and move at your own pace to reach them. For example, instead of saying, "I will be more active," set a goal such as, "I will take a walk after lunch at least two days a week." Ask your family, friends, and coworkers to help you. They can join you, cheer you on, help you get back on track after a setback, and celebrate your successes with you!

No matter what, keep trying. You can do it![1]

Section 14.3 | Making Exercise a Shared Enjoyment

Active people generally live longer and have a lower risk of serious health problems such as heart disease, type 2 diabetes, obesity, and certain cancers. For those with chronic diseases, physical activity can help manage these conditions and reduce complications. About one in two adults lives with a chronic disease, and among those, about half have two or more.

Help your family stay active and have fun while doing it. Consider what your family can do together to be more physically active. Here are some ideas:

MAKE TIME
- **Identify free times**. Keep track of your daily activities for one week. Choose two 30-minute time slots you could dedicate to family activity time.
- **Add physical activity to your daily routine**. For example, walk or bike to work or a friend's house, walk the dog with

---

[1] "Tips to Help You Get Active," National Institute of Diabetes and Digestive and Kidney Diseases (NIDDK), May 2017. Available online. URL: www.niddk.nih.gov/health-information/weight-management/tips-get-active/all-content. Accessed September 7, 2024.

Building an Active Lifestyle

your children, exercise while watching TV, or park farther from your destination.
- **Try walking, jogging, or swimming during your lunch hour, or take fitness breaks instead of coffee breaks.** Do something active after dinner with your family or on weekends.
- **Check out activities that require little time, such as walking, jogging, or stair climbing.**

BRING OTHERS INTO IT
- Ask friends and family to support your efforts.
- Invite them to be active with you.
- Host a party or social event with activities that get people moving, such as dancing or a jump rope contest.
- Exercise with friends.
- Play with your kids or invite them to join you for an exercise video or fitness game.
- Build new friendships with physically active people by joining a group such as the YMCA or a hiking club.

ENERGIZE YOURSELF
- Plan to be active at times during the day or week when you feel most energized.
- Convince yourself that physical activity will boost your energy level if you give it a chance, and then give it a try.

STAY MOTIVATED
- **Plan ahead.** Make physical activity a regular part of your family's schedule. Write it on a family activity calendar.
- **Join an exercise group or class.** Sign your children up for community sports teams or lessons.
- **Choose activities that do not require new skills, such as walking or climbing stairs.**
- **Exercise with friends at a similar skill level.** Create opportunities for your children to be active with their friends.

BUILD NEW SKILLS
- Find a friend who can teach you new skills.
- Take a class to develop new skills, and enroll your children in classes, such as swimming, dancing, or tennis.

USE AVAILABLE RESOURCES
- Choose activities that do not require expensive gear, such as walking, jogging, jumping rope, or doing push-ups.
- Identify affordable, local resources in your area, such as programs through your community center, park or recreation group, or workplace.

MAKE THE MOST OF ALL CONDITIONS
- Develop a set of activities for you and your family that are available regardless of weather, such as indoor cycling, swimming, stair climbing, rope skipping, mall walking, dancing, or indoor active games.
- When the weather is nice, try outdoor activities such as swimming, jogging, walking, or tennis.[1]

---

[1] "Everyday Ideas to Move More," National Heart, Lung, and Blood Institute (NHLBI), February 13, 2013. Available online. URL: www.nhlbi.nih.gov/health/educational/wecan/get-active/activity-plan.htm. Accessed September 7, 2024.

Chapter 15 | **Staying Active and Eating Right**

Eating healthy foods and staying physically active may help you reach and maintain a healthy weight and improve your mood. You may also find that moving more and eating better can help you keep up with the demands of your busy life and be there for the people who depend on you.

HOW MUCH PHYSICAL ACTIVITY DO I NEED?

To maintain or improve your health, aim for 150 minutes per week—or at least 30 minutes on all or most days of the week—of moderate physical activity. Moderate activities are those in which you can talk—but not sing—while doing, such as brisk walking or dancing. These activities speed up your heart rate and breathing.

If you have not been active, work slowly toward the goal of 150 minutes per week. For example, start by doing light or moderate activities for shorter amounts of time throughout the week. You can gain some health benefits even if you do as little as 60 minutes of moderate physical activity per week.

For best results, spread out your physical activity throughout the week. Even 10 or 15 minutes at a time counts, and any amount of physical activity is better than none at all.

To lose weight and keep it off, you may need to be even more active. Aim for 300 minutes per week, or an hour a day 5 days a week. On at least 2 days per week, also include activities that strengthen your muscles. Examples include workouts using hand weights or rubber strength bands.

HOW CAN I EAT HEALTHIER?
A healthy meal includes vegetables, fruits, and small portions of protein and whole grains. These foods provide fiber and important nutrients such as vitamins and minerals. When planning meals for you and your family, consider including:
- a salad or other different-colored vegetables such as spinach; sweet potatoes; and red, green, orange, or yellow peppers
- fat-free or low-fat milk and milk products, or nondairy products such as almond or rice milk
- different-colored fruits, including apples, bananas, and grapes
- lean beef, pork, or other protein foods such as chicken, seafood, eggs, tofu, or beans
- whole grains such as brown rice, oatmeal, whole-wheat bread, and whole-grain cornmeal

Treats are fine if you have them once in a while. Just do not eat foods such as candy, ice cream, or cookies every day. Limit sweet treats to special occasions, and keep portions small. Have one cookie or piece of candy rather than trying every kind.

Remember that alcohol, juices, soda, and other sweet drinks have a lot of sugar and calories.

If you cannot have milk or milk products because you have trouble digesting lactose, the sugar found in milk, try lactose-free milk or yogurt. Besides milk and milk products, you can get calcium from calcium-added cereals, juices, and drinks made from soy or nuts. Eating dark green leafy vegetables such as collard greens and kale and canned fish with soft bones like salmon can also help you meet your body's calcium needs.

HOW CAN I EAT WELL WHEN AWAY FROM HOME?
Here are some ways to make healthy food choices when you are on the go:
- Avoid heavy gravies, salad dressings, or sauces. Leave them off or ask for them on the side so you can control how much you eat.

Staying Active and Eating Right

- Try to avoid fried foods and fast food. Instead of fried chicken, order baked, broiled, or grilled chicken, or a turkey sandwich with whole-grain bread.
- Share a meal with a friend or take half of it home.
- Take healthy snacks with you to work, such as apples or fat-free yogurt with fruit.[1]

SPECIFIC TIPS FOR DIFFERENT FOOD GROUPS
Fruit
Fresh, frozen, or canned fruits are great choices. Try fruits beyond apples and bananas, such as mangoes, pineapples, or kiwis. When fresh fruit is not in season, try a frozen, canned, or dried variety. Be aware that dried and canned fruit may contain added sugars or syrups. Choose canned varieties of fruit packed in water or in its own juice.

Vegetables
Add variety to grilled or steamed vegetables with a herb such as rosemary. You can also sauté vegetables in a nonstick pan with a small amount of cooking spray. Or try frozen or canned vegetables for a quick side dish—just microwave and serve. Frozen peppers, broccoli, or onions can give stews and omelets a quick and convenient boost of color and nutrients.

Look for frozen and canned vegetables without added salt, butter, or cream sauces.

Calcium-Rich Foods
In addition to fat-free and low-fat milk, consider low-fat and fat-free yogurts without added sugars. These come in a variety of flavors and can be a great dessert substitute.

---

[1] "Keep Active & Eat Healthy to Improve Well-Being & Feel Great," National Institute of Diabetes and Digestive and Kidney Diseases (NIDDK), January 2018. Available online. URL: www.niddk.nih.gov/health-information/weight-management/keep-active-eat-healthy-feel-great. Accessed September 6, 2024.

Fortified soy alternatives and canned sardines and salmon are also good sources of calcium. Vitamin D aids in calcium absorption. Sources of vitamin D can include:
- fortified drinks such as milk and fortified soy beverages
- fortified foods such as yogurt or some cereals
- some seafoods

Meats

If your favorite recipe calls for frying fish or breading chicken, try healthier variations by baking or grilling. You might also try dry beans in place of meats. Ask friends or search the Internet and magazines for recipes with fewer calories. You may be surprised to find you have a new favorite dish!

Comfort Foods

You can still enjoy your favorite foods, even if they are high in calories, fat, or added sugars. The key is to eat them only once in a while.

Some general tips for comfort foods:
- **Eat them less often**. If you normally eat these foods every day, cut back to once a week or once a month.
- **Eat smaller amounts**. If your favorite higher-calorie food is a chocolate bar, have a smaller size or only half a bar.
- **Try a lower-calorie version**. Use lower-calorie ingredients or prepare food differently.

For example, a macaroni and cheese recipe might include whole milk, butter, and full-fat cheese. You can try remaking it with nonfat milk, less butter, low-fat cheese, fresh spinach, and tomatoes. Remember not to increase your portion size.

Maintaining a balance between physical activity and healthy eating is essential for a healthy lifestyle. Aim for 150 minutes of moderate activity per week, and choose nutrient-dense foods that provide the energy and nutrients your body needs. Whether at home or on the go, making mindful choices can help you achieve your health goals.[2]

---

[2] "Tips for Healthy Eating for a Healthy Weight," Centers for Disease Control and Prevention (CDC), December 28, 2023. Available online. URL: www.cdc.gov/healthy-weight-growth/healthy-eating. Accessed September 6, 2024.

Chapter 16 | Creating and Sticking to a Fitness Plan

Chapter Contents
Section 16.1—Building Sustainable Exercise Habits 145
Section 16.2—Goal Setting for Physical Activity Success 147

Section 16.1 | Building Sustainable Exercise Habits

Studies have identified several factors linked to better exercise adherence in various groups. Here are five key factors that can help individuals stick to their resolutions throughout the year.

ENJOYMENT

The best type of physical activity is one that is continued regularly. One study found that among previously inactive people with obesity who tried high-intensity functional training, those who enjoyed the exercise at baseline were more likely to stick with it and continue doing similar exercises after the study. Health professionals should encourage individuals to explore various types and combinations of physical activities until they find something they enjoy. People should also feel comfortable exploring different types of physical activity if they become bored with one. It is important to note that the type of exercise or physical activity preferred is not as important as how much time is regularly spent performing that exercise. The *Physical Activity Guidelines for Americans* recommends adults get at least 150 minutes of moderate-to-vigorous aerobic physical activity each week, along with at least two days of muscle-strengthening activity for health benefits.

SELF-EFFICACY

Aside from time and cost, intimidation and lack of knowledge about what to do in a gym are commonly cited as barriers to exercise and reasons for quitting. In a study of people with coronary artery disease, both self-directed motivation and self-efficacy were important determinants of short-term (6-month) exercise adherence. To boost self-efficacy, support from gym staff, a personal trainer, or friends can help build knowledge of exercise techniques and workout structures. People can also seek online resources from certified fitness professionals with instructions, videos, and templates. Group fitness is another way to build self-efficacy. Learning

Fitness and Exercise Sourcebook, Seventh Edition

yoga, weight lifting, cycling, or functional training in a coached group setting can better prepare individuals to be active on their own and feel confident in doing so.

SOCIAL SUPPORT

It is often easier to stick to a habit or behavior when social and family networks are supportive. In a study of 100 middle-aged and older adults, social support—in addition to pain and perceived benefits of exercise—predicted adherence to a 12-month, at-home exercise program. It is important for people to build—and for health professionals to encourage and facilitate—social support for physical activity. This can be achieved by inviting friends and family to join in the new exercise habit and/or seeking out new social opportunities with others who share an interest in the same activities. Health professionals can encourage partner or group workouts or refer individuals to walking or other activity groups in the community. People are more likely to stick with exercise if their friends are involved too.

ACCOUNTABILITY

Along with support, accountability can also be a motivating factor. A qualitative study with a group of middle-aged women indicated that accountability was one of several factors that enabled exercise. Research has shown that people who exercise in groups are more likely to see results. Accountability can be established by working out with a friend, a coach, or a workout partner. Sharing an exercise journey online can also build accountability. For example, posting on social media about going to the gym may increase the likelihood of following through.

INTEGRATION INTO THE DAILY ROUTINE

Lack of time is often cited as a barrier to physical activity, but it does not have to be. Planning ahead is a great way to help overcome this barrier. In the same study of women mentioned earlier, having a daily routine that incorporated physical activity helped enable regular exercise. Health professionals can encourage individuals to

Creating and Sticking to a Fitness Plan

schedule weekly workouts in their calendars to ensure they fit into their daily routines. Workouts can also be broken up into smaller blocks to better fit into the day. For example, someone could spend one hour in the gym or split it into two 30-minute sessions, or even take two 15-minute brisk walks throughout the day.[1]

Having a record will help you stay on track and see your progress.
- Write down what you do every day.
- Start out slowly.
- Aim to reach at least 150 minutes (2½ hours total) per week.
- Try to do strength training at least two days a week.[2]

Section 16.2 | Goal Setting for Physical Activity Success

Adults need to identify benefits of personal value to them. For some people, the health benefits, which are the focus of the *Physical Activity Guidelines for Americans*, are compelling enough to motivate them to be active. For others, different reasons are key motivators for being active. For example, physical activity:
- provides opportunities to enjoy recreational activities, often in a social setting
- improves personal appearance and feelings of energy and well-being
- provides a chance to help a family member or friend be active
- gives older adults a greater opportunity to live independently in the community

---

[1] Office of Disease Prevention and Health Promotion (ODPHP), "5 Factors That Help People Stick to a New Exercise Habit," U.S. Department of Health and Human Services (HHS), January 10, 2018. Available online. URL: https://health.gov/news/blog-bayw/2018/01/5-factors-help-people-stick-new-exercise-habit. Accessed September 6, 2024.
[2] "Make Physical Activity a Habit," National Heart, Lung, and Blood Institute (NHLBI), November 1, 2022. Available online. URL: www.nhlbi.nih.gov/sites/default/files/publications/THT-CHW-PhysicalActivityLog.pdf. Accessed September 6, 2024.

SET PERSONAL GOALS FOR PHYSICAL ACTIVITY

Individuals should set goals for activities that allow them to achieve the benefits they value. When setting goals, people can consider doing a variety of activities and trying both indoor and outdoor activities. Simple goals are fine. For example, a brisk walk in the neighborhood with friends for 45 minutes three days a week and walking to lunch twice a week may be just the right approach for someone who wants to increase both physical activity and social opportunities. More ambitious goals are fine, too. For example, a person may create a physical activity plan aimed at training for a 10-kilometer community run. Multipurpose activities are another way to incorporate physical activity into busy lives. For example, people can use active transportation—walking, biking, or wheelchair walking—to get to school, work, or a store.

DEVELOP KNOWLEDGE AND SKILLS TO ATTAIN GOALS

It is important to learn about the types and amounts of activity needed to attain personal goals. For example, if weight loss is a goal, it is useful to know that vigorous-intensity activity can be more time-efficient in burning calories than moderate-intensity activity. If running is a goal, it is important to learn how to reduce the risk of running injuries by selecting an appropriate training program and proper shoes. If regular walking is a goal, learning about neighborhood walking trails can help attain this goal.[1]

Many people find that having a firm goal in mind motivates them to move forward on a project. Goals are most useful when they are specific, realistic, and important to the individual. Consider both short- and long-term goals. Success depends on setting goals that truly matter. Write down goals, put them where they can be seen often, and review them regularly.

---

[1] Office of Disease Prevention and Health Promotion (ODPHP), "Current Guidelines," U.S. Department of Health and Human Services (HHS), August 24, 2021. Available online. URL: https://health.gov/our-work/nutrition-physical-activity/physical-activity-guidelines/current-guidelines. Accessed September 5, 2024.

Creating and Sticking to a Fitness Plan

SHORT-TERM GOALS

Short-term goals help make physical activity a regular part of daily life. For these goals, think about the things needed to get or do in order to be physically active. For example, walking shoes may be needed to figure out how to fit physical activity into a busy day. Make sure short-term goals will truly help increase activity. Here are a few examples of short-term goals:
- Today, decide to be more active.
- Tomorrow, find out about exercise classes in the area.
- By the end of this week, talk with a friend about exercising together a couple of times a week.
- In the next two weeks, make sure to have the shoes and comfortable clothes needed to start the selected activity.
- By the end of the month, start an exercise class or physical activity.

For those already active, short-term goals can focus on increasing their level of physical activity. For example, over the next week or two, work toward moving at a pace where the conversation becomes a little more challenging, increase the amount of weight lifted, or try a new kind of physical activity. No matter the starting point, reaching short-term goals will increase confidence in progressing toward long-term goals.

LONG-TERM GOALS

After writing down short-term goals, long-term goals can be identified. Focus on where you want to be six months, a year, or two years from now. Long-term goals should be realistic, personal, and important. Here are a few examples of long-term goals:
- By this time next year, swim one mile three times a week.
- In six months, have your blood pressure under control by increasing physical activity and following a doctor's advice.[2]

---

[2] National Institute on Aging (NIA), "Get Fit For Life: Exercise & Physical Activity for Healthy Aging," National Institutes of Health (NIH), January 2024. Available online. URL: https://order.nia.nih.gov/sites/default/files/2024-05/get-fit-life-book.pdf. Accessed September 5, 2024.

Chapter 17 | Strategies for Prompts to Encourage Physical Activity

Prompts such as signs or reminders inform and motivate people to make the choice to be active in specific places. Communities and institutions can use prompts to encourage physical activity in places such as:
- transit stations
- worksites
- universities
- shopping malls
- airports
- walkable community environments

POINT-OF-DECISION SIGNAGE
Motivational signs or other prompts can encourage physical activity, such as taking the stairs instead of elevators or escalators. Signs can remind people of an immediate opportunity to be physically active and provide information about the health benefits of physical activity.

WAYFINDING IN WALKABLE PLACES
Wayfinding helps people walk or use public transit with more confidence by reducing the stress associated with navigating unfamiliar environments. Wayfinding signs placed at strategic points direct

people to nearby destinations, including parks, recreation facilities, and other attractions.[1]

STAIRWELL IDEAS

Taking the stairs instead of an elevator is a good way for people to add physical activity to their day. Modifying stairwells can make them safer and more attractive. Incentives and motivational signs can also be great ways to encourage people to use the stairs.

For maximum health benefits, adults need at least 150 minutes a week of moderate-intensity physical activity. That can be split into 22 minutes a day, 30 minutes each day for five days a week, or whatever works best in one's schedule. Even a few minutes help, including the time it takes to climb the stairs.

To encourage people to take the stairs, building managers can:
- modify stairwells to be safe and attractive
- provide incentives
- post motivational signs

Physical Appearance

Consider these ideas to make stairwells more inviting:
- **Carpet your stairwell if it is not already, or replace carpet that is in poor condition**. Add rubber treading for safety.
- **Paint the walls with bright colors**. If permitted, you can also hang artwork in the stairwell. Other ideas for framed art include cartoons and children's drawings. Change pictures periodically to keep stair users engaged.
- **Create themed stairwells**. For example, transport stair users to a Hawaiian beach or tropical rainforest. You could also create your own cartoon, with a frame or two per floor.

---

[1] "Strategies for Prompts to Encourage Physical Activity," Centers for Disease Control and Prevention (CDC), February 7, 2024. Available online. URL: www.cdc.gov/physical-activity/php/strategies/encouraging-physical-activity.html. Accessed September 9, 2024.

Strategies for Prompts to Encourage Physical Activity

- **Create a catchy rhyme with several lines.** Put the first line of the rhyme on the first floor, the second line on the second floor, and so on. Users would have to travel all the way to the top to read the entire rhyme.
- **Use creative lighting, such as track lighting, incandescent lighting, or halogen lighting.** You could also add an electronic message board and upbeat music appropriate for a workplace.
- **Create a "fitness zone" inside the stairwell.** Start with a sign that says, "You are entering the Fitness Zone."
- **Put numbers on the doors to let users know which floor they are on.** This will also help them track their progress.
- **Allow users to add their signatures to each floor, creating a graffiti wall.**
- **Leave room for motivational signs.**
- **Host a kick-off event with a grand reopening of your improved stairwell.**
- **Commit to maintaining the stairwell so it always looks its best.**

Incentives

Incentives can encourage people to use the stairs. Conduct focus groups to gather information about the signs, colors, and artwork that would motivate people to use the stairs. Use this information to determine what incentives they would appreciate. Keep the incentives within policy and regulations.

Here are some incentive ideas:

- **Map progress.** Make it seem as if users are climbing to a peak, such as Mount Everest or a local landmark. On each flight, show them a "map" of where they are.
- **Hold drawings among stairwell users for prizes, if such incentives are permitted.**
- **Create a challenge.** Ask users to keep track of the number of flights they walk in a week or a month. Award prizes for first, second, and third place. If prizes are not an option, let winners select the music or art in the stairwells for the next week or month.

- **Have a contest for slogans to increase stair use.** These slogans can be incorporated into your artwork and motivational signs. Be sure to note whose slogan is on which sign!

Motivational Signs

Motivational signs can increase awareness of the stair options. For example, hang signs by the elevators saying, "Have you thought of taking the stairs today?" Remind people of the health benefits associated with physical activity. Appeal to environmentally conscious people by pointing out how much energy is used to run an elevator.

You could also add footsteps leading from the elevators to the stairs and have a message spelled out along the way. Or, post arrows showing the way to the stairs.

OTHER IDEAS
Enhance Skills

Help people who want to take the stairs but tire easily or face other barriers. Provide motivation and support for taking the stairs once a day, even for one flight. Help people build up to taking more stairs or taking them more often. Counting the stairs and marking how far people go on the stairs can help build stair-climbing skills.

Provide Opportunities for Trial Behavior

Offer opportunities for people to try using the stairs. Perhaps sponsor a "use the stairs for a day" campaign. You could also reward people for using the stairs for one flight, one day, or one week.

Create a Supportive Social Environment

If your stairwells were unpleasant before your renovation, it may take time to change people's attitudes. Talk about the stairwell positively. By providing users with encouragement, incentives, and messages that support this perception, you can make the stairwell a happy, fun place.[2]

---

[2] "Prompts to Encourage Physical Activity: Stairwell Ideas," Centers for Disease Control and Prevention (CDC), March 7, 2024. Available online. URL: www.cdc.gov/physical-activity/php/stairwell-prompts. Accessed September 9, 2024.

Chapter 18 | Overcoming Obstacles to Physical Activity

Physical activity provides both immediate and long-term health benefits and is one of the best ways to improve your overall health. It is essential for healthy aging, can reduce the effect of chronic diseases, and helps prevent early death. However, common barriers may prevent you from being physically active.

Learn to overcome these barriers and make physical activity a regular part of your day.

LACK OF TIME
- Monitor your daily activities for one week. Identify at least five 30-minute time slots you could use for physical activity.
- Add physical activity to your daily routine. For example, walk or ride your bike to work or while shopping, walk the dog, or take the stairs.
- Organize school activities around physical activity.
- Choose activities such as walking, jogging, or stair climbing that fit the time you have available, even for a few minutes.
- Use physical activity facilities and programs at work.
- Hold walking meetings and conference calls if possible.
- During phone calls, try to stand, stretch, or walk.

LACK OF SOCIAL SUPPORT
- Explain your interest in physical activity to friends and family. Ask for their support.
- Invite friends and family members to be physically active with you.
- Plan social activities that involve physical activity.
- Develop new friendships with physically active people.
- Join a gym or group, such as the YMCA or a hiking club.

LACK OF ENERGY
- Schedule physical activity for times of the day or week when you feel energetic.
- Start slowly and build up to longer durations or more intense activities.

LACK OF MOTIVATION
- Make physical activity a regular part of your daily or weekly schedule, and write it on your calendar.
- Invite a friend to exercise with you regularly and mark it on both your calendars.
- Join an exercise group or class.

FEAR OF INJURY
- Learn how to warm up and cool down properly to prevent injury.
- Learn the best types of exercises for your age, fitness level, skill level, and health status.
- Choose activities you feel you can do safely.
- Gradually increase the amount you do as your confidence and abilities grow.

LACK OF SKILL
- Select activities that do not require new skills, such as walking, climbing stairs, or jogging.
- Take a class to develop new skills.

Overcoming Obstacles to Physical Activity

HIGH COST AND LACK OF FACILITIES
- Select activities that require minimal facilities or equipment, such as walking, jogging, jumping rope, or bodyweight exercises such as pushups or squats.
- Look for inexpensive, convenient resources available in your community, such as park and worksite programs.

WEATHER CONDITIONS
- Develop a set of regular activities that can be done regardless of the weather, such as dancing, indoor swimming, stair climbing, or mall walking.
- Or, bundle up, go outside, and have fun![1]

Table 18.1 offers practical solutions to common barriers to incorporating physical activity into daily lives. Each obstacle, such as lack of time, fatigue, or coordination issues, is paired with actionable strategies to help overcome these challenges and maintain a regular exercise routine.[2]

Table 18.1. Ways to Overcome Obstacles

Obstacle	Try This
I do not have time.	• Monitor your daily activities for one week with this diary. • Find at least three 30-minute time slots you could use for physical activity.
I do not want to do this alone.	• Join a group, such as a class at the YMCA or a hiking club.
I am too tired.	• Schedule physical activity for times in the day or week when you feel energetic. • Add physical activity to your workday by walking during your lunch break and taking the stairs when possible.

---

[1] "Overcoming Barriers to Physical Activity," Centers for Disease Control and Prevention (CDC), April 5, 2024. Available online. URL: www.cdc.gov/physical-activity-basics/overcoming-barriers. Accessed September 9, 2024.
[2] "Steps for Getting Started with Physical Activity," Centers for Disease Control and Prevention (CDC), April 17, 2024. Available online. URL: www.cdc.gov/healthy-weight-growth/physical-activity/getting-started.html. Accessed September 9, 2024.

Table 18.1. Continued

Obstacle	Try This
I have so much to do already.	• Make physical activity a regular part of your schedule by writing it on your calendar.
I will probably hurt myself.	• Ask a health professional what physical activities are right for your age, fitness level, skill level, and health.
I am not coordinated.	• Skip the dance classes that require coordination and choose activities such as walking or biking instead. • Look for online activities to do at home, where it will be OK if you are out of step with the rest of the class.
I cannot learn something new.	• Walk if you are able. • If your mobility is limited, see DeskFit (www.nasa.gov/sites/default/files/atoms/files/hq_deskfit_booklet_6.10.2020.pdf) for ideas of things you can do. • Consider community or online resources for older adults. • Try a variety of activities to find something you can learn.
My job requires me to travel.	• At airports, walk to your gate. • If driving, spend 10 minutes doing physical activity at rest stops. • Find a physical activity you can access on a mobile device wherever you are. • When possible, stay in places with swimming pools or fitness centers and use those facilities. • Take the stairs every time you can.
I am busy with young children.	• Trade babysitting time with a friend, neighbor, or family member who also has small children. When it is their turn to watch the children, it is your turn to be physically active. • As children get older, make physical activity a family event with bike rides or walks.

Chapter 19 | Measuring Health and Fitness

Chapter Contents
Section 19.1—Heart Rate Targets for Fitness 161
Section 19.2—Body Mass Index (BMI) for Health
              Assessment 164
Section 19.3—Energy Balance and Weight Management 168

Section 19.1 | Heart Rate Targets for Fitness

Physical inactivity greatly increases your risk of developing heart disease. Heart disease occurs when the arteries that supply blood to the heart muscle become hardened and narrowed due to a buildup of plaque on the inner walls of the arteries. Plaque is the accumulation of fat, cholesterol, and other substances. As plaque continues to build, blood flow to the heart is reduced.

Heart disease is serious—and often fatal. It is the leading cause of death in the United States, with 500,000 people dying from it each year. Many others with heart problems become permanently disabled. This is why it is vital to take action to prevent heart disease. Regular physical activity should be part of everyone's heart disease prevention plan.

TRACKING YOUR TARGET HEART RATE

As you become more physically active, how will you know if you are improving your heart and lung fitness? The best way is to track your target heart rate during activity. Your target heart rate is a percentage of your maximum heart rate, which is the fastest your heart can beat based on your age. Unless you are in excellent physical condition, any physical activity that raises your heart rate above 75 percent of your maximum rate is likely to be too strenuous. Similarly, an activity that raises your heart rate to less than 50 percent of your maximum provides too little conditioning for your heart and lungs.

GETTING INTO THE ZONE

The most beneficial activity level is between 50 and 75 percent of your maximum heart rate. This range, called your "target heart rate zone," is ideal for improving cardiovascular health. During the first few months of your activity program, aim to reach 50 percent of your maximum rate. As you get in better shape, you can gradually increase this to 75 percent.

Remember that "getting into the zone" does not mean pushing yourself to the limit. For example, while walking briskly or jogging, you should still be able to carry on a conversation. If you cannot,

Fitness and Exercise Sourcebook, Seventh Edition

slow down slightly. A gradual, gentle approach will help you maximize your benefits and minimize your risks.

WHAT IS YOUR NUMBER?

To find your target heart rate zone, refer to Figure 19.1 and locate the age closest to yours. For example, if you are 40, your target zone is 90–135 beats per minute. If you are 53, the closest age on the chart is 55, so your target zone is 83–123 beats per minute. Keep in mind that the figures in the chart are averages, so use them as general guidelines.

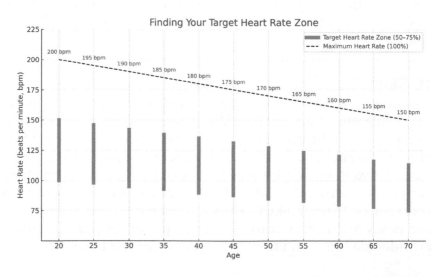

Figure 19.1. Finding Your Target Heart Rate Zone

National Heart, Lung, and Blood Institute (NHLBI)

TAKING YOUR PULSE

To determine if you are within your target heart rate zone, take your pulse immediately after finishing your activity. Here is how:

- **Place the tips of your first two fingers lightly over one of the two blood vessels on your neck, located**

Measuring Health and Fitness

to the left and right of your Adam's apple. Another convenient pulse spot is the inside of your wrist, just below the base of your thumb.
- **Count your pulse for 10 seconds and multiply the result by six.**
- **If your pulse falls within your target zone, your activity is providing good benefits for your heart and lungs.** If it is below your target zone, move a bit faster next time, as long as you are comfortable. If it is above your target zone, slow down. Avoid working at or near your maximum heart rate, as that can be too strenuous.
- **Eventually, you will consistently be engaging in activity within your target zone.** To track your progress, check your pulse after at least one activity session per week.

TIPS FOR HEART HEALTH
- Become—and stay—physically active.
- Balance your calorie intake with the calories you burn through physical activity.
- Lose weight if you are overweight.
- If you smoke, stop. Avoid secondhand smoke whenever possible.
- Control high blood pressure (HBP).
- Control high cholesterol.
- Manage diabetes.
- Choose foods low in saturated fat, *trans* fat, cholesterol, sugar, and salt. Enjoy more fruits, vegetables, and whole grains.[1]

---

[1] "Your Guide to Physical Activity and Your Heart," National Heart, Lung, and Blood Institute (NHLBI), June 2006. Available online. URL: www.nhlbi.nih.gov/files/docs/public/heart/phy_active.pdf. Accessed September 8, 2024.

Section 19.2 | Body Mass Index (BMI) for Health Assessment

Body mass index (BMI) is a simple, reliable, and low-cost measure used to assess health. Having a BMI outside the healthy weight range can increase a person's risk for certain health problems. BMI is interpreted differently for children and adults.

WHY USE BODY MASS INDEX?

Body mass index is a quick, inexpensive, and reliable screening tool for assessing a person's weight relative to height. A BMI outside the healthy weight range increases the risk of certain health problems. For example, people with a BMI in the obesity range have a higher risk of type 2 diabetes, heart disease, and other health issues.

However, BMI is just one measure of health. Health-care providers should also consider other factors, such as physical exams, lab results, and health behaviors, to get a more complete picture of a person's health.

HOW IS BODY MASS INDEX CALCULATED?

Body mass index is a measure of body weight relative to height. The Centers for Disease Control and Prevention (CDC) offers calculators to help you calculate BMI. For children and teens aged 2–19, use the CDC's BMI Calculator for Child and Teen (www.cdc.gov/bmi/child-teen-calculator/index.html). For adults aged 20 and older, use the CDC's Adult BMI Calculator (www.cdc.gov/bmi/adult-calculator/index.html).

To calculate BMI manually, use the following formulas:
- **Metric Units**: weight (kg)/[height (m)]^2
- **Metric Units (cm)**: [weight (kg)/height (cm)/height (cm)] × 10,000
- **U.S. Customary Units**: weight (pounds)/[height (in)]^2 × 703

HOW IS BODY MASS INDEX CALCULATED FOR CHILDREN AND TEENS?
Calculating BMI in children and teens involves these steps:
- Measure the child's height and weight. Refer to Measuring Children's Height and Weight (www.cdc.gov/bmi/child-teen-calculator/measure-child-height-weight.html) for guidance.
- Input the child's height, weight, age, and sex into the CDC's BMI Calculator for Child and Teen (www.cdc.gov/bmi/child-teen-calculator/index.html).

Discuss the results with the child's health-care provider if you have questions or concerns.

HOW DO I INTERPRET BODY MASS INDEX PERCENTILES FOR CHILDREN AND TEENS?
Health-care providers use percentiles to evaluate growth patterns in children and teens. A child's or teen's BMI percentile reflects their BMI in comparison to a reference population of the same age and sex. This reference population is used to create CDC's BMI-for-Age Growth Charts (www.cdc.gov/growthcharts/cdc-growth-charts.htm).

For example, a seven-year-old girl with a BMI in the 88th percentile has a BMI equal to or higher than 88 percent of seven-year-old girls in the reference population. This places her in the overweight category, defined as a BMI between the 85th and 95th percentile for her age and sex.

HOW IS BODY MASS INDEX INTERPRETED FOR ADULTS?
To interpret BMI for adults (20 years and older), use standard BMI categories, regardless of age, sex, or race. For example, an adult who is 5 feet 8 inches tall and weighs 200 pounds has a BMI of 30.4, which falls into the obesity category (a BMI of 30.0 or higher).

SHOULD I INTERPRET BODY MASS INDEX THE SAME WAY FOR CHILDREN AND ADULTS?

No. BMI is interpreted differently for children and teens than for adults. Since children and teens are still growing, their BMI is compared to others of the same age and sex using BMI-for-age percentiles and the CDC's BMI-for-Age Growth Charts (www.cdc.gov/growthcharts/cdc-growth-charts.htm).

HOW IS BODY MASS INDEX USED TO ASSESS OBESITY?

For adults (20 years or older), enter your height and weight into the CDC's Adult BMI Calculator (www.cdc.gov/bmi/adult-calculator/index.html) to find your BMI and BMI category. For adults, obesity is defined as a BMI of 30.0 or higher. Speak to your health-care provider about your BMI and its relation to your risk of chronic diseases.

For children and teens (ages 2–19), use the CDC's Child and Teen BMI Calculator (www.cdc.gov/bmi/child-teen-calculator/index.html). The tool will calculate BMI, BMI percentile, and BMI category. You can also view the results on a growth chart. For children and teens, obesity is defined as a BMI at or above the 95th percentile for sex and age. Discuss your child's BMI with their health-care provider to understand how it may relate to their overall health.

WHAT ARE THE HEALTH CONSEQUENCES OF OBESITY FOR CHILDREN AND TEENS?

Obesity during childhood or adolescence is linked to various physical and mental health conditions, including:
- high blood pressure (HBP)
- high cholesterol, high triglycerides, and other abnormal lipids
- prediabetes and type 2 diabetes
- respiratory conditions, such as asthma and sleep apnea
- mental health conditions, such as depression and anxiety
- low self-esteem and low self-reported quality of life (QOL)

WHAT ARE THE HEALTH CONSEQUENCES OF OBESITY FOR ADULTS?

Adults with obesity are at increased risk for several health problems, including:
- high blood pressure and high cholesterol
- type 2 diabetes
- stroke
- many types of cancer
- severe illness from coronavirus 2019 (COVID-19)
- mental health conditions, such as depression and anxiety
- joint problems, such as osteoarthritis
- breathing problems, such as asthma and sleep apnea

IS BODY MASS INDEX A GOOD INDICATOR OF BODY FAT?

For most people, BMI is a good indicator of whether they have too much or too little body fat. However, BMI does not directly measure body fat, nor can it distinguish fat mass from lean body mass (muscle and bone). Additionally, BMI does not show where fat is distributed in the body.

BMI is moderately to strongly associated with other measures that do capture the amount, type, and distribution of fat. A health-care provider can help evaluate a person's health risks related to their BMI and body fat.

IF AN ATHLETE OR SOMEONE WITH A LOT OF MUSCLE HAS A HIGH BODY MASS INDEX, ARE THEY STILL CONSIDERED OVERWEIGHT?

Based solely on BMI, people with significant muscle mass may have a BMI in the overweight (BMI of 25.0–29.9) or obesity (BMI of 30.0 or more) categories. However, BMI cannot distinguish between fat, muscle, and bone mass, which all affect weight.

BMI is just one indicator of health. For a more complete assessment, health-care providers should consider other factors, such as medical history, health behaviors, physical exams, and lab results.[1]

---

[1] "BMI Frequently Asked Questions," Centers for Disease Control and Prevention (CDC), June 28, 2024. Available online. URL: www.cdc.gov/bmi/faq. Accessed September 8, 2024.

Section 19.3 | Energy Balance and Weight Management

WHAT IS ENERGY BALANCE?
Energy is another word for "calories." Your energy balance is the comparison of calories consumed through eating and drinking to calories burned through physical activity. What you eat and drink is "energy in." What you burn through physical activity is "energy out."

You burn a certain number of calories just by breathing and digesting food. You also burn calories ("energy out") through your daily routine. For example, children burn calories just by being students—walking to their lockers, carrying books, and so on—and adults burn calories by walking to the bus stop, shopping, and so on.

An important part of maintaining energy balance is the amount of "energy out" (physical activity) that you do. People who are more physically active burn more calories than those who are less active.

- The same amount of "energy in" (calories consumed) and "energy out" (calories burned) over time = weight stays the same.
- More "in" than "out" over time = weight gain.
- More "out" than "in" over time = weight loss.

Your "energy in" and "energy out" do not need to balance every day. Achieving a balance over time will help you maintain a healthy weight in the long term. Children also need to balance their energy, but their growth should also be considered.

Energy balance in children occurs when the amount of "energy in" and "energy out" supports natural growth without promoting excess weight gain.

ESTIMATED CALORIE REQUIREMENTS
Table 19.1 presents estimated amounts of calories needed to maintain energy balance (and a healthy body weight) for various gender and age groups at three different levels of physical activity. The estimates are rounded to the nearest 200 calories and were determined using an equation from the Institute of Medicine (IOM).

Measuring Health and Fitness

Table 19.1. Estimated Calorie Requirements (in Kilocalories) for Each Gender and Age Group at Three Levels of Physical Activity

		Activity Level		
Gender	**Age (Years)**	**Sedentary**	**Moderately Active**	**Active**
Child	2–3	1,000	1,000–1,400	1,000–1,400
Female	4–8	1,200	1,400–1,600	1,400–1,800
Female	9–13	1,600	1,600–2,000	1,800–2,000
Female	14–18	1,800	2,000	2,400
Female	19–30	2,000	2,000–2,200	2,400
Female	31–50	1,800	2,000	2,200
Female	51+	1,600	1,800	2,000–2,200
Male	4–8	1,400	1,400–1,600	1,600–2,000
Male	9–13	1,800	1,800–2,200	2,000–2,600
Male	14–18	2,200	2,400–2,800	2,800–3,200
Male	19–13	2,400	2,600–2,800	3,000
Male	31–50	2,200	2,400–2,600	2,800–3,000
Male	51+	2,000	2,200–2,400	2,400–2,800

Source: U.S. Dietary Guidelines for Americans.

- These levels are based on Estimated Energy Requirements (EER) from the IOM Dietary Reference Intakes macronutrients report (2002), calculated by gender, age, and activity level for reference-sized individuals. "Reference size," as determined by IOM, is based on median height and weight for ages up to 18 and median height and weight for that height to give a body mass index (BMI) of 21.5 for adult females and 22.5 for adult males.
- "Sedentary" means a lifestyle that includes only the light physical activity associated with typical day-to-day life.
- "Moderately active" means a lifestyle that includes physical activity equivalent to walking about 1.5–3 miles per day at 3–4 miles per hour, in addition to the light physical activity associated with typical day-to-day life.
- "Active" means a lifestyle that includes physical activity equivalent to walking more than 3 miles per day at 3–4 miles per hour, in addition to the light physical activity associated with typical day-to-day life.
- The calorie ranges shown are to accommodate the needs of different ages within the group. For children and adolescents, more calories are needed at older ages, and for adults, fewer calories are needed at older ages.

ENERGY BALANCE IN REAL LIFE

Think of it as balancing your "lifestyle budget." For example, if you know you and your family will be attending a party where you might eat more high-calorie foods than usual, you may want to consume fewer calories for a few days before to balance it out. Alternatively, you can increase your physical activity level a few days before or after the party to burn off the extra energy.

The same applies to your children. If they will be attending a birthday party and eating cake and ice cream—or other foods high in fat and added sugar—help them balance their calories the day before and/or after by encouraging them to be more physically active.

Here is another way to consider energy balance in real life:

Eating just 150 calories more per day than you burn can lead to a gain of 5 pounds over six months. That is a gain of 10 pounds per year. If you want to avoid this weight gain or lose the extra weight, you can either reduce your "energy in" or increase your "energy out." Doing both is the best way to achieve and maintain a healthy body weight.

Here are some ways to cut 150 calories (energy in):
- Drink water instead of a 12-ounce regular soda.
- Order a small serving of French fries instead of a medium, or choose a salad with dressing on the side.
- Eat an egg-white omelet (with three eggs) instead of whole eggs.
- Use tuna canned in water (6-ounce can) instead of oil.

Here are some ways to burn 150 calories (energy out) in just 30 minutes (for a 150-pound person):
- Shoot hoops.
- Walk two miles.
- Do yard work (gardening, raking leaves, etc.).
- Go for a bike ride.
- Dance with your family or friends.[1]

---

[1] "Balance Food and Activity," National Heart, Lung, and Blood Institute (NHLBI), February 13, 2013. Available online. URL: www.nhlbi.nih.gov/health/educational/wecan/healthy-weight-basics/balance.htm. Accessed September 9, 2024.

Chapter 20 | Choosing Fitness Partners

Chapter Contents
Section 20.1—Supporting Loved Ones in Staying Active 173
Section 20.2—Family Fitness through Fun and
 Engaging Activities 175

Chapter 20 | Choosing Fitness Partners

Section 20.1 | Supporting Loved Ones in Staying Active

Regular physical activity is good for everyone's health! Physical activity is anything that gets your body moving.

Aim for at least 150 minutes of moderate-intensity aerobic activity each week. In addition, do activities that strengthen your muscles at least two days a week.

If you have not been active before or for a while, start slowly. Even five minutes of physical activity has real health benefits! Once you get the hang of it, add a little more activity each time.

WHAT KINDS OF ACTIVITY SHOULD I DO?

To get all the health benefits of physical activity, do a combination of aerobic and muscle-strengthening activities.

- **Aerobic activities make you breathe harder and get your heart beating faster.** Walking fast is an example of moderate-intensity aerobic activity, and jogging or running is an example of vigorous-intensity aerobic activity.
- **Muscle-strengthening activities make your muscles stronger.** Examples include lifting weights, using resistance bands, and doing body-weight exercises such as push-ups.

WHAT ARE THE BENEFITS OF PHYSICAL ACTIVITY?

Physical activity increases your chances of living longer. It can also help:

- control your blood pressure, blood sugar, and weight
- lower your "bad" cholesterol and raise your "good" cholesterol
- prevent heart disease, type 2 diabetes, and some types of cancer

And that is not all. Being more active can:

- boost your mood
- help you sleep better

- make your bones, muscles, and joints healthier
- lower your chances of becoming depressed
- lower your risk of falls and reduce arthritis pain
- help you have fun and feel better about yourself[1]

If someone you care about is having a hard time getting active, you can help. Here are some tips to get you started:

SUGGEST ACTIVITIES YOU CAN DO TOGETHER
- **Start small**. Try taking a walk together after dinner twice a week or doing push-ups during commercials while watching TV.
- **Mix it up**. Find different ways to move, such as dancing or doing balance exercises.
- **Try something new**. Take a fitness class together or play a sport you both enjoy.

MAKE IT PART OF YOUR REGULAR ROUTINE
- Meet up at the local park or recreation center on your way home from work.
- Wake up a bit earlier, so you can go for a brisk walk together before breakfast.
- Pick a set time for physical activity, like right after your favorite TV show.
- Ride your bike or walk to the store or coffee shop.

TAKE TIME TO UNDERSTAND THE SITUATION
What are your loved one's reasons for not being more active? For example, they might feel overwhelmed or embarrassed. Talk about what is making it difficult to get physical activity—then ask what you can do to be supportive.

---

[1] Office of Disease Prevention and Health Promotion (ODPHP), "Get Active," U.S. Department of Health and Human Services (HHS), August 16, 2024. Available online. URL: https://health.gov/myhealthfinder/health-conditions/diabetes/get-active. Accessed September 8, 2024.

Choosing Fitness Partners

RECOGNIZE SMALL EFFORTS
- **Be patient.** Change takes time.
- **Remember.** Any amount of physical activity is better than none!
- **Offer encouragement and praise.** Say: "Great job getting a walk in today!"
- **Point out positive choices.** Say: "I'm glad we're walking to the park instead of driving."[2]

Section 20.2 | Family Fitness through Fun and Engaging Activities

According to the *Physical Activity Guidelines for Americans*, children need 60 minutes or more of moderate-to-vigorous intensity physical activity daily, and adults require at least 150 minutes of moderate intensity activity per week to maintain or improve overall health and reduce the risk of chronic disease.

Physical activity is one of the most important things families can do to improve their health. When families engage in physical activity together, they not only benefit from being and growing together but also build healthy habits for the future.

It is never too late to start a family fitness journey. With a few creative changes, an active lifestyle can be achieved. Here are some ideas to get you and your family moving.

INDOOR ACTIVITIES
- **Play active games.** Create an indoor obstacle course, play charades, hide-and-seek, complete a scavenger hunt, or build a fort.

---

[2] Office of Disease Prevention and Health Promotion (ODPHP), "Help a Loved One Get More Active: Quick Tips," U.S. Department of Health and Human Services (HHS), February 14, 2024. Available online. URL: https://health.gov/myhealthfinder/health-conditions/diabetes/help-loved-one-get-more-active-quick-tips. Accessed September 8, 2024.

Fitness and Exercise Sourcebook, Seventh Edition

- **Embrace modern technology**. Many online services offer free virtual fitness classes and activity games that can be played on your TV or tablet.
- **Turn up the tunes**. Play musical chairs, freeze dance, or have a dance party while doing indoor chores.
- **Break up sitting time**. Plan an instant recess with light exercises such as jumping jacks, squats, push-ups, sit-ups, marching in place, or Hula-Hoop.

OUTDOOR ACTIVITIES
- **Pound the pavement**. Walk or run outside, hike, or explore trails at a local park. If you have a pet, take family walks with your dog.
- **Put wheels to the ground**. Ride a bicycle, skateboard, rollerblade, or scooter on a bike path, in an empty parking lot, or through your neighborhood.
- **Encourage backyard games**. Play tag, Frisbee, jump rope, Hula-Hoop, or hopscotch.
- **Assign active chores**. Mow the lawn, rake leaves, weed the garden, or wash the car—chores can be active, too!
- **Have a ball**. Play soccer or tennis, toss a baseball or football, or enroll children in organized sports.
- **Make a splash**. Run through sprinklers, jump over waves at the beach, paddle in a lake, try paddleboarding, or have a water balloon fight.[1]

EXPLORING TEAM AND INDIVIDUAL SPORTS
Parents can encourage their children to try both team and individual sports. Traditional team sports such as soccer, baseball, and basketball are great for introducing physical activity, but there is also a growing trend toward non-traditional or individual sports that can become lifelong activities. Participating in a variety of

---

[1] "Family Fitness," U.S. Department of Homeland Security (DHS), May 5, 2021. Available online. URL: www.dhs.gov/employee-resources/blog/2021/05/05/family-fitness. Accessed September 8, 2024.

Choosing Fitness Partners

sports throughout childhood increases the likelihood of continued activity in adulthood. Local parks, the YMCAs, and other organizations often offer classes and lessons in various sports and fitness activities, with free trials or family discounts to make participation more accessible.

Sample activities include:
- biking
- rowing
- dance
- golf
- group exercise classes (e.g., barre, kickboxing, boot camp, Zumba)
- parkour (e.g., obstacle courses)
- rock climbing
- running
- skateboarding
- swimming
- yoga

Some children are motivated by tracking their activity. Technology can be integrated with apps that record physical activity or with simple pedometers or fitness trackers.

EXPLORING INDEPENDENT AND FAMILY PHYSICAL ACTIVITIES

Independent physical activities to recommend include walking the dog, using exercise playing cards, desk cycles, fitness videos, or fitness equipment such as resistance bands, steps, or free weights. Parents know what motivates their children and can build on that knowledge.

Research and experience confirm that children, especially adolescents, are more likely to try something new when they are with friends. Involving a peer group in physical activity increases the likelihood of ongoing participation.

Family vacations provide great opportunities to try new activities, whether paddleboarding at the beach, mountain biking, or exploring a park or playground. Even small, fun activities such as kicking a ball in the yard, having a dance party in the kitchen, or hosting a family push-up contest can make a big difference. Children will love whatever fitness activities they do with their families.

Family-based fitness is more likely to become lifelong fitness, offering countless physical, cognitive, and social benefits.[2]

---

[2] Office of Disease Prevention and Health Promotion (ODPHP), "Promoting Family Fitness," U.S. Department of Health and Human Services (HHS), April 25, 2018. Available online. URL: https://health.gov/news/blog-bayw/2018/04/promoting-family-fitness. Accessed September 8, 2024.

Chapter 21 | Roles and Responsibilities of Fitness Trainers and Instructors

Fitness trainers and instructors work with people of all ages and skill levels. They lead, instruct, and motivate individuals or groups in exercise activities, including cardiovascular workouts (for heart and blood circulation), strength training, and stretching.

PERSONAL FITNESS TRAINERS

Exercise trainers, also known as "personal fitness trainers," work with individual clients or small groups. They may train in a gym or in clients' homes. They evaluate their clients' current fitness levels, personal goals, and skills. Based on this evaluation, they develop personalized training programs for their clients to follow and monitor their progress. In gyms or other fitness facilities, these trainers often sell training sessions to members.

GROUP FITNESS INSTRUCTORS

Group fitness instructors organize and lead group exercise classes, which may include cardiovascular exercises, muscle strengthening, or stretching. Some instructors create routines or select exercises for participants to follow and choose appropriate music to accompany the movements. Others teach pre-choreographed routines developed by fitness companies or organizations. They may lead classes that use specific exercise equipment, such as stationary bicycles, teach a specific conditioning method, such as yoga, or instruct specific age groups, such as seniors or youths.

Fitness and Exercise Sourcebook, Seventh Edition

CORE RESPONSIBILITIES OF FITNESS TRAINERS AND INSTRUCTORS

Fitness trainers and instructors typically perform the following duties:
- Demonstrate or explain how to perform various exercises and routines to minimize injuries and improve fitness.
- Observe clients to ensure they are using the correct technique during exercises.
- Provide modifications during workouts to help clients feel successful.
- Monitor clients' progress and adapt programs as needed.
- Explain and enforce safety rules and regulations related to sports, recreational activities, and exercise equipment use.
- Provide clients with information or resources on topics such as nutrition and lifestyle.
- Administer emergency first aid if needed.

ADDITIONAL RESPONSIBILITIES BEYOND FITNESS

Fitness trainers and instructors work with individual clients or prepare and choreograph their own group classes. In addition to their fitness duties, they may perform other tasks, such as managing the front desk, signing up new members, giving tours of the facility, or supervising the weight-training and cardiovascular equipment areas. Fitness trainers and instructors may also promote their facilities and instruction through social media, by writing newsletters or blog posts, or by creating posters and flyers.[1]

---

[1] U.S. Bureau of Labor Statistics (BLS), "Fitness Trainers and Instructors," U.S. Department of Labor (DOL), April 17, 2024. Available online. URL: www.bls.gov/ooh/personal-care-and-service/fitness-trainers-and-instructors.htm#tab-2. Accessed September 8, 2024.

Chapter 22 | Debunking Weight Loss Myths and Scams

It would be nice if you could lose weight simply by taking a pill, wearing a patch, or rubbing in a cream, but claims that you can lose weight without changing your habits are simply untrue. Some of these products could even harm your health.

SPOT FALSE PROMISES
Dishonest advertisers will say just about anything to get you to buy their weight loss products. Here are some of the false promises often seen in weight loss ads:
- Lose weight without dieting or exercising. (You will not.)
- You do not have to watch what you eat to lose weight. (You do.)
- If you use this product, you will lose weight permanently. (Wrong.)
- To lose weight, all you have to do is take this pill. (Not true.)
- You can lose 30 pounds in 30 days. (Nope.)
- This product works for everyone. (It does not.)
- Lose weight with this patch or cream. (You cannot.)

Here is the truth:
- Any promise of miraculous weight loss is simply untrue.
- There is no magic way to lose weight without a sensible diet and regular exercise.

Fitness and Exercise Sourcebook, Seventh Edition

- No product will let you eat all the food you want and still lose weight.
- Permanent weight loss requires permanent lifestyle changes, so do not trust any product that promises once-and-for-all results.
- U.S. Food and Drug Administration (FDA)-approved fat-absorption blockers or appetite suppressants do not result in weight loss on their own. These products must be used in conjunction with a low-calorie, low-fat diet, and regular exercise.
- Products promising lightning-fast weight loss are always a scam. Worse, they can ruin your health.
- Even if a product could help some people lose weight in certain situations, there is no one-size-fits-all product guaranteed to work for everyone. Everyone's habits and health concerns are unique.
- Nothing you can wear or apply to your skin will cause you to lose weight.

FITNESS AND WEIGHT LOSS PRODUCTS

Using an electronic muscle stimulator alone will not work. You might have seen ads for electronic muscle stimulators claiming they will help you lose weight or get rock-hard abs. However, according to the FDA, while these devices may temporarily strengthen, tone, or firm a muscle, they have not been shown to help you lose weight or achieve six-pack abs.

If you decide to join a gym, make sure you know what you are agreeing to. Not all gym contracts are the same, so before you commit, read the contract and confirm that it includes everything the salesperson promised. Also, find out if there is a "cooling-off" or trial period, and check the cancellation policy. Do you get a refund if you cancel? You can also look for reviews online from other clients to help you decide if you want to join that particular gym.

Home exercise equipment can be a great way to shape up, but only if you use it regularly. Some exercise equipment ads promise that you can shape up and lose weight quickly and without much effort. The truth is that to get the benefits of exercise, you have to do the work. If you decide to buy exercise equipment for your home, first check online reviews to see what other customers' experiences have been. Also, find out the real cost of the equipment. Some companies advertise "three easy payments of $49.99," but you must consider taxes, shipping, and any subscription or other fees required to make the equipment work.

RECOGNIZE FAKE STORIES ONLINE

Scammers place false stories online through fake news websites, blogs, banner ads, and social media to sell their weight loss products. For example, they create so-called news reports about how an ingredient—such as garcinia cambogia or gonji—found in a diet pill is supposedly effective for weight loss. However, there is no new discovery. The stories are false.

Know that:
- Scammers often use stolen logos of real news organizations, or they use names and web addresses that resemble those of well-known news websites. They may even add public photos of reporters to make you think the report is real.
- Scammers write glowing online reviews themselves, pay others to do it, or cut and paste positive comments from other fake sites.
- Scammers use images showing dramatic weight loss, but these images are just stock or altered photographs, not photos of people who actually used the product they want you to buy.

OTHER THINGS TO WATCH OUT FOR

"Free" trial offers are often not free at all. Many people who have signed up for "free" trials for weight loss products have ended up paying a lot of money and have been billed for recurring shipments they did not want. The FDA has found tainted weight loss products. In recent years, the FDA has discovered hundreds of dietary supplements that contain potentially harmful drugs or other chemicals not listed on the product label. Many of these products are for weight loss and bodybuilding.[1]

---

[1] "The Truth Behind Weight Loss Ads," Federal Trade Commission (FTC), July 2022. Available online. URL: https://consumer.ftc.gov/articles/truth-behind-weight-loss-ads. Accessed September 8, 2024.

Part 4 | Categories of Exercise or Physical Fitness

Chapter 23 | Aerobic Activity

HOW MUCH IS ENOUGH?
As little as 60 minutes a week of moderate-intensity aerobic activity, such as walking briskly, helps your heart. For major health benefits, aim for at least 150 minutes a week. Or go for 75 minutes a week of more vigorous activity, such as playing basketball, running, or jumping rope, which provides the same benefits. The bottom line: more activity means a bigger boost to your health. It is up to you how you reach your personal targets. For example, 30 minutes of physical activity five times a week is one option if you are aiming for 150 minutes a week.[1]

AEROBIC ACTIVITIES
Aerobic activities, also called "endurance activities," increase your breathing and heart rates. These activities help keep you healthy, improve your fitness, and help you perform daily tasks. Aerobic activities improve the health of your heart, lungs, and circulatory system. They can also delay or prevent many diseases, such as diabetes, colon and breast cancers, and heart disease. Physical activities that build endurance include:
- brisk walking or jogging
- yard work (mowing, raking)
- dancing
- swimming

---

[1] "Move More: Making Physical Activity Routine," National Heart, Lung, and Blood Institute (NHLBI), 2022. Available online. URL: www.nhlbi.nih.gov/sites/default/files/publications/HM-2022-MoveMoreFactSheet_508.pdf. Accessed September 9, 2024.

- biking
- climbing stairs or hills
- playing tennis or basketball

Build up to at least 150 minutes of activity a week that makes you breathe hard. To reach this goal, try to be active throughout your day and avoid sitting for long periods of time.

SAFETY TIPS
- Do a little light activity, such as easy walking, before and after your aerobic activities to warm up and cool down.
- Listen to your body: aerobic activities should not cause dizziness, chest pain or pressure, or a feeling like heartburn.
- Be sure to drink liquids when doing any activity that makes you sweat. If your doctor has told you to limit your fluids, be sure to check before increasing the amount you drink while exercising.
- If you are exercising outdoors, be aware of your surroundings.
- Dress in layers so you can add or remove clothes as needed for hot and cold weather.
- To prevent injuries, use safety equipment, such as a helmet when bicycling.[2]

WORKING TOGETHER FOR HEALTH
While aerobic activities benefit the heart the most, aerobic, strength training, and flexibility exercises are all vital components of a comprehensive physical activity program. They work together in important ways. For example, resistance exercises help build the muscle strength, balance, and coordination needed for aerobic activities. Flexibility training, on the other hand, helps you move

---

[2] National Institute on Aging (NIA), "Four Types of Exercise Can Improve Your Health and Physical Ability," National Institutes of Health (NIH), January 29, 2021. Available online. URL: www.nia.nih.gov/health/exercise-and-physical-activity/four-types-exercise-can-improve-your-health-and-physical. Accessed September 9, 2024.

Aerobic Activity

your muscles and joints more easily and reduces the risk of injury during aerobic exercises. Many activities that promote flexibility and strength are also relaxing and enjoyable.

THREE MOVES FOR HEALTH

While not usually aerobic, the activities below offer numerous health benefits and are enjoyable ways to get and stay in shape. All are offered at many YMCAs, community or recreation centers, and gyms.

- Yoga is a system of physical postures, stretching, and breathing techniques that can improve flexibility, balance, muscle strength, and relaxation. Many styles are available, ranging from slow and gentle to athletic and vigorous. A recent study found that regular yoga practice may help to minimize weight gain in middle age.
- Tai chi is an ancient Chinese practice based on shifting body weight through a series of slow movements that flow rhythmically together into one graceful gesture. This gentle, calming practice can help improve flexibility and balance and gradually build muscle strength.
- Pilates is a body conditioning routine that seeks to strengthen the body's "core" (torso), usually through a series of mat exercises. Another Pilates method uses special exercise machines, which are available at some health clubs. The practice can strengthen and tone muscles and increase flexibility.[3]

FIND WAYS TO STAY MOTIVATED

Think about ways to remain active once you start. Some ideas include:
- Get active with a friend.
- Choose your favorite activities.
- Do activities in short chunks of time.

---

[3] "Your Guide to Physical Activity and Your Heart," National Heart, Lung, and Blood Institute (NHLBI), June 2006. Available online. URL: www.nhlbi.nih.gov/files/docs/public/heart/phy_active.pdf. Accessed September 9, 2024.

Reap the benefits of physical activity by:
- being healthier
- increasing your chances of living longer
- sleeping better
- reducing stress

Even when you are really busy, find ways to be active, like walking during your lunch break at work.[4]

---

[4] "Be Active for a Healthy Heart," National Heart, Lung, and Blood Institute (NHLBI), January 21, 2018. Available online. URL: www.nhlbi.nih.gov/sites/default/files/publications/14-5202.pdf. Accessed September 9, 2024.

Chapter 24 | Martial Arts for Youth

HOW TO PLAY
Martial arts—a special type of defense skill—originated in East Asia. Today, they are taught worldwide for self-defense and conflict avoidance. As a form of physical activity, martial arts emphasize body and mind control, discipline, and confidence. There are many martial arts styles, but since certain types put more strain on the joints (such as the knees) than others, here are some of the best options for kids your age:

- **Judo comes from Japan and means "gentle way."** It is similar to Jujitsu, one of the oldest martial arts, but not as intense. Judo involves many wrestling moves and teaches participants how to make good decisions and be mentally strong. Judokas (judo players) focus on competition.
- **Karate comes from Japan and means "empty hand."** It is Japan's most popular martial art. Karate uses feet, legs, elbows, head, and fists for kicking, punching, defensive blocks, and more. Karate emphasizes defense and sometimes incorporates weapons.
- **Tae Kwon Do comes from Korea and means "the way of the foot and fist."** It is famous for high kicks. Tae Kwon Do became Korea's national sport in 1955 and is now the world's most popular martial art.

Other martial arts include:
- Aikido
- Hwarang Do

Fitness and Exercise Sourcebook, Seventh Edition

- Kung Fu
- Jujitsu
- Kendo
- Ninjutsu
- Northern and Southern Shaolin Boxing
- Tai Chi
- T'an Su Do

GEAR UP

Most martial arts students wear white pants, a white jacket, and a cloth belt. For some martial arts, the belt color indicates the student's skill level and personal development—from white (beginner) to black (expert). The colors represent nature. For example, the white belt that students start with symbolizes a seed. The yellow belt, which they receive next, represents the sunshine that helps the seed grow. To advance from one grade level to another, students must pass several tests—5 for the green belt, 9 for the brown belt, and 10 for the black belt! You can earn a first-degree black belt in two to four years, but even then, there is still more to learn—there are 10 black belt levels!

For sparring (practice fighting), wear full gear, including a mouthpiece and padding for your head, hands, feet, and shins.

PLAY IT SAFE

Look for an instructor who emphasizes respect and discipline but also has plenty of patience. The class area should be spacious and have a smooth, flat floor with padding. The fewer students in the class, the better—more attention for you!

Wear all the appropriate gear. Warm up and stretch so you are loose and ready to go. You need proper instruction before attempting any moves. And once you learn the moves, remember your limits. For example, white belt students should not spar (practice fight).

When you are ready for matches, make sure you have an instructor nearby to supervise. Some martial artists use special weapons (such as swords), but unless you are highly advanced, using them is almost guaranteed to lead to injury—so, no weapons. During

Martial Arts for Youth

your match, make sure your partner knows when you are ready to stop. If you let your guard down, your partner might see it as an opportunity to take you down!

FUN FACTS
- If you open your hands wide and shove something, your force spreads across your palm and fingers. But if you hold all of your fingers together and hit with only the side of your hand or fingertips, the same amount of force is concentrated on a smaller area, making the hit harder. Try this on yourself to feel the difference—just do not overdo it!
- In karate competitions, opponents are not allowed to actually hit each other. Their moves must stop just short of contact.
- The original five Chinese fighting styles we call Kung Fu mimic the movements of tigers, cranes, leopards, snakes, and dragons.
- Judo was the first martial art accepted at the Olympic Games. 197 countries participate![1]

---

[1] "Martial Arts Activity Card," Centers for Disease Control and Prevention (CDC), May 9, 2015. Available online. URL: www.cdc.gov/healthyschools/bam/cards/martialarts.html. Accessed September 9, 2024.

Chapter 25 | Aquatic Exercise

Chapter Contents
Section 25.1—Benefits and Safety of Water-Based Exercise.....197
Section 25.2—Swimming Risks and Safety Measures 198

Section 25.1 | Benefits and Safety of Water-Based Exercise

Water-based exercise provides both physical and mental health benefits, particularly for people with chronic conditions such as diabetes, heart disease, and arthritis. However, recreational water can also spread illness or cause injury, so it is essential to know how to protect yourself and others.

HEALTH BENEFITS

Swimming can improve mood, and many people report enjoying water-based exercise more than exercising on land. People can also exercise longer in water without increased joint or muscle pain, making it especially helpful for those with arthritis or osteoarthritis. Water-based exercise can improve the use of arthritic joints, reduce pain, and avoid worsening symptoms. In particular, people with rheumatoid arthritis have shown more significant health improvements after participating in hydrotherapy (exercise in warm water) than in other activities.

For people with fibromyalgia, swimming can reduce anxiety, and exercise therapy in warm water can alleviate depression and improve mood. Parents of children with developmental disabilities report that recreational activities, such as swimming, strengthen family connections.

Water-based exercise also benefits older adults by enhancing their quality of life (QOL) and reducing disability. It can help improve or maintain bone health, particularly for post-menopausal women.

STAYING HEALTHY AND SAFE WHILE YOU SWIM

Understanding how to prevent illness and injury in or around the water is important for staying healthy and safe while swimming.

You can contract swimming-related illnesses if you swallow, have contact with, or inhale mist from water contaminated with germs. The most common swimming-related illnesses include diarrhea, skin rashes, swimmer's ear, pneumonia or flu-like illness, and irritation of the eyes or respiratory tract.

KEEPING POOLS SAFE AND CLEAN

Maintaining clean and germ-free pools is essential for providing healthy swimming experiences for all swimmers. Responding quickly to contamination events in pools, whether caused by animals or humans, is critical.

Animals can carry germs that contaminate pool water, so it is important to take precautions when animals have been in or near the pool.

Many germs that cause swimming-related illnesses, such as *Cryptosporidium* and *Giardia*, are spread through fecal matter in the water. Vomit, especially if it contains previously eaten food, can also introduce illness—causing germs. Both fecal matter and vomit should be cleaned up immediately from pool water and surrounding surfaces.[1]

Section 25.2 | Swimming Risks and Safety Measures

STAYING SAFE AND HEALTHY DURING SWIMMING AND WATER ACTIVITIES

Swimming and other recreational water activities come with health and safety risks, such as swimming-related illnesses and drowning.

Swimming-related illnesses are diseases caused by germs in the water where people swim and play. Drowning is the leading cause of death for children aged one to four and the second leading cause of unintentional injury death for kids aged 5–14. Natural bodies of water such as oceans, lakes, and rivers can pose additional hazards. Knowing the safety and quality of those waters before visiting is important.

---

[1] "Swimming and Your Health," Centers for Disease Control and Prevention (CDC), May 8, 2024. Available online. URL: www.cdc.gov/healthy-swimming/about. Accessed September 9, 2024.

Aquatic Exercise

Learning how to reduce the risk of injury and illness from the water you swim in can help you and your loved ones maximize all the health benefits that swimming can bring.[1]

The most common swimming-related illnesses include diarrhea, skin rashes, swimmer's ear, pneumonia or flu-like symptoms, and irritation of the eyes or respiratory tract.

You can get swimming-related illnesses if you swallow, have contact with, or inhale mists of water contaminated with germs. You can also contract these illnesses from exposure to chemicals in the water or by inhaling chemicals that evaporate and turn into gas in the air.

Diarrhea outbreaks are the most common swimming-related illness outbreaks. People who are sick with diarrhea can spread germs to others if they have an accident in the water. If others swallow the contaminated water, they can become infected. While chemicals such as chlorine or bromine can inactivate most germs in properly treated water within minutes, *Cryptosporidium* can survive for more than seven days.

RISK FACTORS

Children, pregnant individuals, and people with weakened immune systems are at the highest risk for swimming-related illnesses.

Recreational water may be contaminated with *Cryptosporidium*, which can cause life-threatening symptoms in people with weakened immune systems. These individuals should consult their health-care provider before participating in water activities such as swimming.

HOW TO PREVENT SWIMMING-RELATED ILLNESSES

Pools, hot tubs, and water playgrounds that maintain proper chlorine or bromine levels and pH are less likely to spread germs. Injuries and drownings are less likely when trained staff and adequate safety equipment are present.

---

[1] "Guidelines for Healthy and Safe Swimming," Centers for Disease Control and Prevention (CDC), May 14, 2024. Available online. URL: www.cdc.gov/healthy-swimming/safety/index.html. Accessed September 9, 2024.

Before You Get In
- Check the latest inspection results on the state or local health department website or on-site.
- Make sure the drain at the bottom of the deep end is visible, and check that drain covers are secured and in good condition.
- Look for lifeguards:
  - If on duty, lifeguards should be focused on swimmers, not distracted.
  - If no lifeguard is present, locate safety equipment such as a rescue ring or pole.
- Ensure no chemicals are left out in the open.

Check Yourself
- Stay out of the water if you have diarrhea. If you have been diagnosed with *Cryptosporidium*, avoid swimming until two weeks after your diarrhea has completely stopped.
- Avoid swimming if you have an open cut or wound, especially from surgery or piercing. If you must enter the water, use waterproof bandages to cover the wound completely.
- Shower before swimming. A quick one-minute rinse removes most dirt or anything else on your body that could deplete the chlorine or bromine needed to kill germs.

Once You Are In
- Do not pee or poop in the water.
- Do not swallow the water.
- Use well-fitting, Coast Guard-approved life jackets for flotation support, not air-filled toys such as water wings.
- Keep an eye on children at all times. Kids can drown in seconds, and drowning often occurs in silence.
- Take children on bathroom breaks and check diapers every hour.
- Dry ears thoroughly after swimming.[2]

---

[2] "Preventing Swimming-Related Illnesses," Centers for Disease Control and Prevention (CDC), May 14, 2024. Available online. URL: www.cdc.gov/healthy-swimming/prevention/index.html. Accessed September 9, 2024.

Chapter 26 | Walking and Hiking

Chapter Contents
Section 26.1—Enhancing Physical Activity and Health
through Walking 203
Section 26.2—Hiking with Friends and Family 205

Section 26.1 | Enhancing Physical Activity and Health through Walking

WALKING AND PHYSICAL ACTIVITY

More than 145 million adults now include walking as part of their physically active lifestyle. Over 6 in 10 people walk for transportation, fun, relaxation, exercise, or activities such as walking the dog. The percentage of people who reported walking at least once for 10 minutes or more in the previous week increased from 56 percent in 2005 to 62 percent in 2010.

Physical activity helps control weight but also provides other health benefits. Walking can improve health even without weight loss. People who are physically active live longer and have a lower risk of heart disease, stroke, type 2 diabetes, depression, and some cancers. Creating safe spaces to walk can help more people become physically active.

KEY FACTS ABOUT WALKING AND PHYSICAL ACTIVITY
The Physical Activity Gap among Adults

- Adults need at least 150 minutes of aerobic physical activity per week at a moderate level, such as brisk walking, for at least 10 minutes at a time.
- Women and older adults are less likely to meet the recommended weekly physical activity levels.
- Inactive adults have a higher risk of:
  - early death
  - heart disease
  - stroke
  - type 2 diabetes
  - depression
  - cancers
- Regular physical activity helps people maintain a healthy weight.
- Walkable communities encourage more physical activity.

Fitness and Exercise Sourcebook, Seventh Edition

Factors Influencing Walking
- The West and Northeast regions have the highest percentage of adults who walk, but the South showed the largest increase in adults walking compared to other regions.
- More adults with arthritis or high blood pressure (HBP) are now walking, although this increase has not been seen among adults with type 2 diabetes.
- Walking has increased among adults aged 65 and older, though less so than in other age groups.

The Importance of Safe and Accessible Walking Spaces
- People are more likely to walk when they feel safe from traffic, crime, and other hazards.
- Maintaining surfaces can help prevent falls and make walking easier for those using wheelchairs or strollers, as well as for people with poor vision.
- People need to be aware of safe and convenient places to walk in their communities.
- Walking routes in and near neighborhoods encourage walking to public transportation stops, such as buses, trains, and trolleys.

PRACTICAL WAYS INDIVIDUALS CAN CONTRIBUTE
- Start a walking group with friends and neighbors.
- Help others walk more safely by driving the speed limit and yielding to pedestrians.
- Use crosswalks and crossing signals; avoid jaywalking.
- Participate in local planning efforts to identify ideal sites for walking paths and sidewalks.
- Work with parents and schools to encourage children to walk to school, where it is safe to do so.[1]

---

[1] "More People Walk to Better Health," Centers for Disease Control and Prevention (CDC), August 8, 2012. Available online. URL: www.cdc.gov/vitalsigns/pdf/2012-08-vitalsigns.pdf. Accessed September 9, 2024.

Walking and Hiking

- Make walking fun by going to places you enjoy, such as shopping centers or parks.
- Bring a friend to chat with, or listen to music—just keep the volume low enough to stay aware of your surroundings.

Consider safety as you plan your walks. Walk with others when possible, and bring a phone and ID. Let someone know your walking time and route. If walking after dark, wear a reflective vest or brightly colored clothing. Always be aware of your surroundings.[2]

Section 26.2 | **Hiking with Friends and Family**

Hiking with your friends or family is a great way to enjoy the outdoors, breathe fresh air, and stay active. It is easy to get started—just look for a trail in a national park near you!

Before heading out on your hike, get in shape by walking around your neighborhood with a pack loaded with 5 pounds more gear than you plan to carry. If that goes well, plan a short hike to test your abilities on the trail. For your first day hike (hiking for a day or less without camping overnight), choose a safe, well-marked trail without too many steep climbs to avoid getting tired too soon. Each time you go hiking, challenge yourself by going a little farther and trying a slightly steeper trail.

GEAR UP

Start by investing in a good pair of shoes and thick socks designed for hiking. You can begin with sturdy sneakers with thick soles, but once you tackle more difficult trails, consider hiking boots that fit well. Additionally, get a backpack or fanny pack for your supplies. Dress in layers, and bring a waterproof jacket with a hood in case

---

[2] *NIH News in Health*, "The Benefits of Walking," National Institutes of Health (NIH), March 2016. Available online. URL: https://newsinhealth.nih.gov/2016/03/benefits-walking. Accessed September 9, 2024.

of rain. Do not forget a hat, sunscreen, and sunglasses—the higher you hike, the stronger the sun's rays become.

To ensure a fun and safe hiking experience, always be prepared for unexpected challenges, such as finding the trail if you get lost or encountering bad weather. Bring a map of the area you are hiking in and a sturdy compass. If you do not know how to use a compass, take some time to learn. Carry plenty of water and extra food, such as sports bars or trail mix, in case you have to stay out longer than expected. Adults on your hike should carry waterproof matches and a multipurpose knife. A flashlight and extra batteries are essential for finding your way if you end up hiking after dark. Finally, pack a first aid kit in case of injury.[1]

SAFETY TIPS FOR HIKING

- Stay on marked trails.
- Do not hike alone. Let the slowest person in your group set the pace, especially when children are involved.
- Leave your itinerary with a friend or family member and check in with them when you return.
- Develop an emergency plan before starting your trip. Ensure everyone knows what to do if they get lost or if a medical emergency arises. Give children whistles and instruct them to "stop and blow" if they get lost.
- Take frequent rests or adjust your pace to maintain energy.
- Drink plenty of water, even on cool or wet days, and do not consume your entire supply between refills.
- Wear appropriate clothing, including broken-in, comfortable hiking boots.
- Consider using a hiking pole or walking stick for balance on uneven or hazardous terrain.
- Be mindful of your surroundings and plan your approach before hiking through hazardous areas, especially wet surfaces, which can be dangerous on slopes.

---

[1] "Hiking Activity Card," Centers for Disease Control and Prevention (CDC), May 9, 2015. Available online. URL: www.cdc.gov/healthyschools/bam/cards/hiking.html. Accessed September 9, 2024.

Walking and Hiking

- Consider what to do if you start to slide or fall, and be prepared.
- If you are falling, avoid trying to catch yourself with your hands, elbows, or knees. Landing on your side is safer.
- If you know you are going to slide, lower your center of gravity by sitting down and sliding on your feet or bottom.
- If sliding while standing, keep your weight over your feet and bend your knees—avoid leaning back or forward.

ESSENTIAL ITEMS FOR A DAY HIKE

Extra weight can wear you down and reduce agility on uneven terrain. Pack as lightly as possible, but consider bringing these essentials:
- map
- sunglasses and a hat
- sunscreen
- flashlight
- waterproof matches
- first aid kit
- water and water-purifying tablets
- high-energy bars, granola, candy, or fruit
- extra clothing—temperatures can drop dramatically, especially with elevation changes (For every 1,000 feet of elevation gain, the temperature often drops 3–5 degrees.)[2]

---

[2] U.S. Forest Service (USFS), "Hiking," U.S. Department of Agriculture (USDA), December 27, 2019. Available online. URL: www.fs.usda.gov/visit/know-before-you-go/hiking. Accessed September 9, 2024.

Chapter 27 | Bicycling

Chapter Contents
Section 27.1—Bicycling Basics 211
Section 27.2—Bicycling Safety...212

Section 27.1 | **Bicycling Basics**

Bicycling, or biking, can be a great competitive sport as well as a fun activity to enjoy with friends. There are many types of bicycling to match different personalities. If you love speed, bicycle racing might be your style. If you prefer rugged terrain, mountain biking could be for you. If you simply enjoy pedaling for fun, any type of bicycling will do. Try riding to school or a friend's house!

Biking works on several parts of the body, including the heart, lungs, upper legs, and lower legs.

GEAR UP
- Mountain bikes are strong, stable, and built for gravel roads and tricky trails.
- Racing bikes are designed for speed on pavement, while sport bikes, a combination of both, are versatile for different uses.
- Make sure your helmet fits properly—it should sit just above your eyebrows and be tightly buckled to prevent slipping while riding.

PLAY IT SAFE
Always wear a helmet when riding, as it is required by law in many states. Look for helmets approved by the Consumer Product Safety Commission (CPSC) or Snell B-95 standards, which are best for bicycling. Avoid riding at night or in bad weather, and wear brightly colored or reflective clothes so you can be easily seen. You can even add reflectors or cool reflective stickers to your bike for extra safety and style. Also, be careful of loose pant legs and shoelaces, which can get caught in the bike chain.

BE STREET SMART
Ride on the right side of the road, with traffic, and obey all traffic signs and signals. Discuss the safest routes with your parents to determine the best places to ride near your home.

At intersections, always stop and look left, right, and then left again before proceeding. Use hand signals to indicate turns, and watch out for rough pavement so you can avoid it. While it may be tempting to listen to your favorite tunes, never wear headphones when riding a bike.

FUN FACTS

- The faster you go, the longer it will take to stop once you hit the brakes. If you are going 20 mph and hit the brakes, it will take 15 feet to stop on dry pavement and 23.5 feet on wet pavement—so brake early!
- 100 calories can power a cyclist for three miles, but would only power a car for 280 feet.
- In 1995, 50-year-old Fred Rompelberg set a new speed record for cycling at 166.9 mph.[1]

Section 27.2 | Bicycling Safety

Americans are increasingly bicycling (biking) for commuting, exercise, or recreation. In many states, bicycles are considered vehicles when operated on the road, and bicyclists must follow the same rules.

WEARING A HELMET

Every bike ride should start with putting on a helmet, and ensuring a proper fit is equally important for protection.

Since helmet sizes vary by manufacturer, follow the steps for proper fitting. Although it may take time to adjust the straps, your safety is worth it. Using a mirror or having someone help can make adjustments easier.

---

[1] "Bicycling Activity Card," Centers for Disease Control and Prevention (CDC), May 9, 2015. Available online. URL: www.cdc.gov/healthyschools/bam/cards/bicycling.html. Accessed September 9, 2024.

Choosing a Bicycle Helmet
When selecting a bike helmet, ask yourself these three questions:
- **Is it legit?** Only some helmets meet federal safety standards. Look for a label showing the helmet complies with U.S. Consumer Product Safety Commission (CPSC) standards for safety. Properly used, these helmets protect against skull fractures and severe brain injuries.
- **Does it fit?** A poorly fitting helmet will not protect your skull in a crash. It should be comfortable, sit level on your head, provide adequate coverage without blocking vision, and be snug when fastened.
- **What type is it?** Different helmets are made for specific activities. Choose a helmet designed for bicycling, as it is built to protect against effects associated with riding.

Fitting a Bicycle Helmet
- **Two-finger V at your ears**. Form a V with two fingers around your ear. Adjust the helmet straps to follow this path for both ears.
- **Two fingers under your chin**. When the straps are fastened, you should be able to fit two fingers between the straps and your chin. Adjust as needed to ensure a snug fit without being too tight.

AVOIDING CRASHES
There are two main types of crashes: falls, which are the most common, and collisions with cars, which are the most serious. Regardless of the type of crash, prevention is key. Here are some important bicycle safety facts:
- Bicyclist deaths are highest between June and September.
- Nearly three-quarters of all bicyclist deaths occur in urban areas.

Fitness and Exercise Sourcebook, Seventh Edition

- Failing to yield the right of way and lack of visibility are leading causes of fatal crashes.

BEING PREPARED

- Ride a bike that fits you—riding a bike that is too big makes it harder to control.
- Ensure your bike is in good working condition, especially the brakes.
- Wear equipment to protect yourself and enhance visibility, including a bike helmet, bright clothing during the day, and reflective gear with a white front light and red rear light for nighttime or low-visibility conditions.
- Ride with both hands on the handlebars unless signaling a turn.
- Carry items in a backpack or secure them to the back of the bike.
- Tuck in and tie your shoelaces and pant legs to prevent them from getting caught in the bike chain.
- Plan your route, choosing roads with less traffic and slower speeds. Bike lanes or paths away from traffic are often the safest option.

RIDING DEFENSIVELY

Defensive riding means being alert to traffic and road conditions. Anticipate what others may do before they do it. The sooner you notice a potential conflict, the quicker you can act to avoid a crash.

- Ride with the flow of traffic.
- Obey street signs, signals, and road markings as if you were driving a car.
- Assume other drivers do not see you. Be aware of hazards such as toys, pebbles, potholes, grates, and train tracks.
- Avoid distractions such as texting or listening to music that can take your eyes, ears, or mind off the road.

Bicycling

RIDING PREDICTABLY
Riding predictably helps motorists know your intentions, reducing the risk of a crash.
- Ride where you are expected to be seen, in the same direction as traffic. Use hand signals and look over your shoulder before changing lanes or turning.
- Avoid riding on sidewalks, as cars do not expect traffic there. If sidewalk riding is necessary, follow these guidelines:
  - Check local laws to ensure sidewalk riding is legal.
  - Watch for pedestrians and pass with care, announcing "on your left" or ringing a bell.
  - Ride in the same direction as traffic. If the sidewalk ends, you will already be moving with traffic.
  - Slow down and be prepared to stop when crossing streets, and follow pedestrian signals.
  - Watch for cars backing out of driveways or turning at intersections.

IMPROVING YOUR RIDING SKILLS
Just as driving a vehicle safely requires practice, so does riding a bike in traffic. Start by practicing in a safe environment away from traffic, such as a park or bike path.

Take an on-bike class offered by your school, local recreation department, or a bike advocacy group. Experience and learning how to navigate and communicate with other drivers, bicyclists, and pedestrians can help build confidence in traffic.

SHARING THE ROAD WITH BICYCLISTS
Drivers need to be aware of cyclists and treat them with the same care as other vehicles on the road.
- Yield to bicyclists as you would to motorists.
- In parking lots or at stop signs, always check your surroundings for other vehicles, including bicycles.
- When turning right on red, look to your right and behind you to avoid hitting a cyclist.

- Obey the speed limit and reduce speed when road conditions warrant.
- Give cyclists room when passing. Do not pass too closely—wait until it is safe to move into an adjacent lane.[1]

---

[1] "Bicycle Safety," National Highway Traffic Safety Administration (NHTSA), April 24, 2010. Available online. URL: www.nhtsa.gov/road-safety/bicycle-safety. Accessed September 9, 2024.

Chapter 28 | Strength and Resistance Training

Chapter Contents
Section 28.1—Basics of Resistance Training................................219
Section 28.2—Strength Training for Healthier Aging...............221

Section 28.1 | Basics of Resistance Training

WHAT IS RESISTANCE TRAINING?
Resistance training, or strength training, is defined as any exercise that causes muscles to contract against an external resistance with the expectation of increases in strength, endurance, or size. Strength training can not only help build strength and muscle but also boost metabolism and aid in managing weight. Resistance training can be a great way to maximize performance and prepare for any task. Physical fitness and activity are crucial to ensuring strength, agility, power, and speed. Adding resistance training to your regimen can improve your performance.

BENEFITS OF RESISTANCE TRAINING
- Strength training is a fundamental part of physical fitness. To develop the strength you need, perform strength training two to three times per week using all seven major muscle groups.
- Resistance training increases bone density and is important for long-term bone health, making individuals tougher and more resistant to injury.
- Strength training improves body composition by reducing fat and increasing muscle.
- Women gain strength from resistance training but do not typically add bulk due to much lower testosterone levels than men. Females can improve their strength without worrying about excessive muscle bulk.
- Balanced strength training helps reduce the risk of overuse injuries, such as tendonitis. Ensure you are working all major muscle groups, not just the "mirror muscles" that are most visible.
- If you are considering taking dietary supplements with your weight training, check Operation Supplement Safety at the Human Performance Resources by Champ website (www.hprc-online.org/resources-partners/opss).

TYPES OF EFFECTIVE RESISTANCE TRAINING
- weight machines at a gym or in a home setup
- free weights such as dumbbells, barbells, kettlebells, and medicine balls
- elastic resistance bands or straps for "suspension training"
- bodyweight resistance training such as pushups, pullups, lunges, and squats
- some kinds of challenging yoga and gymnastic strength moves

STRENGTH TRAINING BASICS
- Working out just two to three days per week using a whole-body program effectively builds strength and muscle.
- Resistance training can use different kinds of weights (dumbbells, barbells, kettlebells, etc.), resistance bands, medicine balls, or body weight.
- Rest muscle groups for about 48 hours between workouts. Get seven to eight hours of sleep to maximize recovery and improvement.[1]

LIFTING WEIGHTS SAFELY
Get started building muscle safely by following these tips:
- **Start slowly, especially if you have not been active for a long time.** Gradually increase your activity level and intensity.
- **Pay attention to your body.** Exhaustion, sore joints, or muscle pain may indicate that you are overdoing it.
- **Use small amounts of weight to start.** Focus on your form, and add more weight gradually over time.
- **Use smooth, steady movements to lift weights into position.** Avoid jerking or thrusting weights.

---

[1] "Performance Triad: The Total Army Family Guide," U.S. Government Publishing Office, August 10, 2012. Available online. URL: www.govinfo.gov/content/pkg/GOVPUB-D101-PURL-gpo65572/pdf/GOVPUB-D101-PURL-gpo65572.pdf. Accessed September 9, 2024.

Strength and Resistance Training

- **Avoid "locking" your arm and leg joints in a straight position.**
- **Do not hold your breath during strength exercises.** Holding your breath can cause changes in your blood pressure. Breathe out as you lift the weights and breathe in as you relax.
- **Ask for help.** To get started, schedule a session or two with a personal trainer, or look for a group class at a local gym, recreation center, or senior center.

Resistance training offers a wide range of benefits, from improving strength and endurance to boosting bone health. By incorporating resistance training into your fitness regimen, you can enhance your overall performance, prevent injuries, and maintain a healthy body composition. Start slowly, ensure proper form, and seek professional guidance if necessary to maximize results safely.[2]

Section 28.2 | Strength Training for Healthier Aging

THE IMPORTANCE OF STRENGTH TRAINING FOR HEALTHY AGING

Strength training builds healthier bodies as we age, with many people performing incredible feats of strength and endurance well into their retirement years. The great news is that you do not have to bench press 300 pounds or run a marathon to enjoy the benefits of strength training.

National Institute on Aging (NIA)-supported researchers have studied the effects of strength training for more than 40 years and identified multiple ways it benefits older adults, including maintaining muscle mass, improving mobility, and increasing healthy years of life.

---

[2] *NIH News in Health*, "Maintain Your Muscle," National Institutes of Health (NIH), March 1, 2020. Available online. URL: https://newsinhealth.nih.gov/2020/03/maintain-your-muscle. Accessed September 9, 2024.

Age-related mobility limitations are a reality for many older adults. Studies show that about 30 percent of adults over age 70 experience difficulty with walking, getting up from a chair, or climbing stairs. In addition to making everyday tasks challenging, mobility limitations are linked to higher rates of falls, chronic disease, nursing home admission, and mortality.

A significant factor contributing to the loss of physical abilities as we grow older is the age-related loss of muscle mass and strength, called "sarcopenia." Muscle mass and strength typically increase steadily from birth and peak between ages 30 and 35. After that, muscle power and performance decline gradually at first, but faster after age 65 for women and 70 for men. These findings come from NIA's Baltimore Longitudinal Study of Aging (BLSA), the longest-running study of human aging, which developed the Short Physical Performance Battery (SPPB) to track mobility and muscle performance. The SPPB measures balance, walking speed, and the ability to rise from a chair five times, rating individuals on a scale from 0 to 4.

While the average decline in strength and power with age is inevitable, it can be substantially slowed by maintaining an active lifestyle. Although it is impossible to "stop the clock," many older adults can increase muscle strength with exercise, which helps maintain mobility and independence.

TYPES OF STRENGTH TRAINING

Strength training, also known as "resistance training," differs from aerobic exercises such as running, cycling, or walking. Weightlifting, using machines or free weights, is one type of resistance training. Other forms include exercises using medicine balls, resistance bands, or bodyweight exercises such as pushups, squats, or yoga. Resistance training involves muscle contraction to lift a heavy object against gravity.

During resistance training, the more weight you lift, the faster your body burns through reserves of adenosine triphosphate (ATP), a molecule that delivers energy to cells. As you lift weights or perform other challenging exercises, your ATP reserves are replenished through a complex metabolic process that sparks short-term chemical changes in the DNA of muscle tissue, making it more attuned to proteins supporting sugar and fat metabolism.

STRENGTH TRAINING FOR OLDER ADULTS WITH OBESITY

While strength training benefits otherwise healthy older adults, it is also effective for those who are overweight or living with obesity. NIA-supported researcher Dennis T. Villareal, MD, a professor at Baylor College of Medicine, found that incorporating weightlifting into an exercise and diet program for older adults with obesity yields better results than diet or aerobic exercise alone.

"Resistance training is the most important component because it builds muscle and reduces muscle loss," he said. "As the relationship between body mass and muscle becomes more positive, participants lose more fat than muscle, improving relative sarcopenia significantly. Combining the two types of exercise had additive effects, so they were better together than separate."

Villareal and his team have observed positive changes in participants who stick with the program. Some volunteers have even exceeded the 10 percent body weight loss target, losing up to 20 percent. The combination of fat loss and muscle gain leads to improved mobility and independence, making participants feel better. Villareal emphasizes the importance of starting slowly and attending regular group classes to build confidence and social connections.

TIPS FOR STAYING STRONG AS WE AGE

There is no denying that our ability to respond to exercise diminishes as we age. Even professional athletes who compete into their 40s do not respond to exercise the same way at age 70 as they did at 30. Here are some realistic tips to stay strong and active as we age:
- **Know what to expect.** Do not compare yourself to younger individuals. Everyone ages differently.
- **Move mindfully.** Exercises incorporating mindfulness with balance and movement, such as tai chi and yoga, can improve strength and help prevent falls and fractures.

- **Make it part of your daily routine.** Walk around the house or office, walk to the store, or take brief exercise or stretching breaks every 15–20 minutes, engaging all muscle groups.
- **Keep it fun.** Exercise does not have to involve running or going to the gym. Activities such as dancing, gardening, or housework count as exercise.
- **Set realistic goals.** Everyone is different, and there is no one-size-fits-all approach.

Strength training offers significant benefits for older adults, including maintaining muscle mass, improving mobility, and increasing healthy years of life. By incorporating resistance exercises into daily routines, individuals can slow the effects of aging, remain independent, and improve their overall quality of life (QOL).[1]

---

[1] National Institute on Aging (NIA), "How Can Strength Training Build Healthier Bodies as We Age?" National Institutes of Health (NIH), June 30, 2022. Available online. URL: www.nia.nih.gov/news/how-can-strength-training-build-healthier-bodies-we-age. Accessed September 9, 2024.

Chapter 29 | Flexibility

THE IMPORTANCE OF FLEXIBILITY IN PHYSICAL FITNESS
The role of flexibility in physical fitness has been debated since the 1950s, and studies have shown inconsistent results when measuring flexibility outcomes with physical activities. That being said, few clinicians would argue against the benefits of maintaining range of motion to perform daily activities effectively. Moreover, some studies show reasonable benefits from stretching, particularly in the context of age-related loss of functionality and managing chronic illnesses.

While more research is needed regarding the specific role of flexibility in overall physical fitness and health, most experts agree that structured flexibility exercises improve general health. Preliminary studies suggest that flexibility may reduce arterial stiffening, which could theoretically reduce cardiovascular disease rates. Stretching may also improve heart rate variability, reduce resting heart rate, and lower blood pressure. Finally, flexibility exercises have consistently demonstrated benefits in both short-term and long-term balance performance.

Current research suggests that warm-up stretching does not immediately reduce the risk of athletic injuries. However, regular stretching over weeks appears to have a long-term benefit in improving muscle power and force, which can positively affect athletic performance. Some studies have also shown a correlation with fewer work-related injuries when stretching is done regularly in the workplace. Additionally, certain medical conditions such as osteoarthritis and adhesive capsulitis often warrant special attention to flexibility training to preserve or regain function and reduce discomfort.

Despite inconsistencies in current research on flexibility training, being able to move the body through a wider range of movements provides more options for accomplishing tasks, enjoying recreational activities, and expressing oneself. When flexibility increases, so do the possibilities for movement.

FACTORS INFLUENCING FLEXIBILITY

Several factors contribute to a person's tendency to be more flexible or stiff. Females tend to be more flexible than males, and flexibility generally declines with age. Various genetic conditions, such as Marfan syndrome and other connective tissue disorders, affect flexibility. Joint hypermobility and joint hypermobility syndrome are two overlapping and somewhat poorly understood conditions associated with pronounced flexibility. These conditions exist on a continuum of severity, affect up to 30 percent of the population, and exhibit a strongly heritable risk pattern.

High degrees of flexibility achieved at a young age may be maintained into adulthood. For example, athletes and artists who exhibit high degrees of flexibility, such as gymnasts and contortionists, typically begin flexibility training at a young age. Long-term conditioning through training and habit undoubtedly contributes to long-term flexibility differences.

COMMON FLEXIBILITY TESTS AND THEIR USES

Although the sit-and-reach test primarily focuses on hamstring extensibility (and is not a reliable measure of lumbar flexibility), it has been used worldwide as a basic instrument for measuring baseline flexibility. Other measures of flexibility include the zipper test, which evaluates shoulder flexibility, and the sitting-rising test, which may also predict overall mortality risk.

RECOMMENDATIONS FOR STRETCHING AND FLEXIBILITY EXERCISES

The American College of Sports Medicine recommends that healthy adults perform stretching exercises at least two days per week, spending about one minute on each major muscle-tendon group (shoulder girdle, chest, neck, trunk, lower back, hips, posterior and anterior legs, and ankles) for about 10 minutes per session. Many

Flexibility

studies have noted benefits in improving the range of motion in joints with just 10–30 seconds of regular stretching. Current literature does not consistently suggest immediate benefits from performing static or dynamic stretching before exercise but warming up with light aerobic activity and stretching is still recommended due to the long-term benefits.

There are many forms of exercise and physical activity that emphasize flexibility. The following is a short list to consider recommending to those interested in improving their flexibility:

- **Yoga**. Research supports the use of yoga to increase flexibility.
- **Pilates**. Research also supports Pilates for increasing flexibility.
- **Massage**. Many types of massage aim to maintain the flexibility of joints and soft tissues.
- **Tai chi**. This inner martial art embodies the ideal of strength with flexibility and has consistently been observed to improve flexibility.
- **Other martial arts**. These often explicitly work to develop flexibility.
- **Dance**. Dance, in many forms around the world, is a fun way to stay flexible.
- **Gardening**. Historically, humans have been bending, squatting, and kneeling for horticulture.
- **Housework**. Depending on how it is done, housework can be an excellent way to exercise the ability to stretch, bend, and reach.[1]

INCORPORATING STRETCHING INTO YOUR ROUTINE

Stretching can increase your freedom of movement to do both the things you need and the things you enjoy. Always warm up your body with some light activity before stretching. It is also beneficial

---

[1] "Pump Up Your Physical Activity," U.S. Department of Veterans Affairs (VA), June 27, 2019. Available online. URL: www.move.va.gov/docs/veteranworkbook/movewbm09.pdf. Accessed September 9, 2024.

Fitness and Exercise Sourcebook, Seventh Edition

to stretch after strength or cardio activities. You should stretch every day, but if that is not possible, aim for at least three times a week for 20 minutes per session.[2]

---

[2] "Improving Flexibility," U.S. Department of Veterans Affairs (VA), May 31, 2024. Available online. URL: www.va.gov/WHOLEHEALTHLIBRARY/tools/improving-flexibility.asp. Accessed September 9, 2024.

Chapter 30 | Mind-Body Exercises

Chapter Contents
Section 30.1—Exploring Mind and Body Practices 231
Section 30.2—Yoga for Health and Wellness 233
Section 30.3—Tai Chi and Qigong 237
Section 30.4—Meditation and Mindfulness 241

Section 30.1 | **Exploring Mind and Body Practices**

MIND AND BODY PRACTICES

Mind and body practices are a large and diverse group of procedures or techniques administered or taught by a trained practitioner or teacher. Examples include acupuncture, massage therapy, meditation, relaxation techniques, spinal manipulation, tai chi, and yoga.

Research findings suggest that several mind and body practices are helpful for a variety of conditions. A few examples include:
- Acupuncture may help ease chronic pain, such as low-back pain, neck pain, and osteoarthritis/knee pain. It may also help reduce the frequency of tension headaches and prevent migraine headaches.
- Meditation may help reduce blood pressure, symptoms of anxiety and depression, and symptoms of irritable bowel syndrome (IBS), as well as flare-ups in people with ulcerative colitis. It may also benefit people with insomnia.
- Tai chi appears to help improve balance and stability, reduce back pain and knee osteoarthritis pain, and improve quality of life (QOL) in people with heart disease, cancer, and other chronic illnesses.
- Yoga may benefit general wellness by relieving stress, supporting good health habits, and improving mental and emotional health, sleep, and balance. Yoga may also help with low-back and neck pain, anxiety or depressive symptoms associated with difficult life situations, quitting smoking, and QOL for people with chronic diseases.

Safety Considerations for Mind and Body Practices

Mind and body practices generally have good safety records when performed by a trained professional or taught by a well-qualified instructor. However, just because a practice is safe for most people does not necessarily mean it is safe for you. Your medical conditions or other special circumstances (such as pregnancy) may affect the safety of a mind and body practice. When considering these practices, ask about the training and experience of the practitioner or teacher, and discuss your individual needs. Also, do not use a mind and body practice to postpone seeing a health-care provider for a health problem.[1]

COMPLEMENTARY HEALTH PRACTICES AMONG CHILDREN AND TEENS

According to a national survey, nearly 12 percent of children and teens (about one in nine) in the United States are using some form of complementary health product or practice, such as chiropractic or spinal manipulation, yoga, meditation, or massage therapy. Mind and body practices include a variety of procedures and techniques done or taught by a trained practitioner or teacher to help improve health and well-being. Older children and teens can do some mind and body activities on their own (or with help from a parent or guardian), such as relaxation techniques and deep breathing. Mind and body practices are generally safe if used appropriately, but the number of studies examining their safety specifically for children is limited.

Safety Considerations for Complementary Health Practices in Children

- Acupuncture appears to be safe for most children, but side effects can occur if performed by poorly trained practitioners.
- Massage therapy has few risks when done by a trained practitioner, but extra precautions are necessary for children with certain health conditions, such as bleeding disorders.
- Relaxation techniques are generally safe for healthy children, though rare cases suggest they might worsen symptoms in children with epilepsy, certain psychiatric conditions, or a history of abuse or trauma.

---

[1] "Mind and Body Practices," National Center for Complementary and Integrative Health (NCCIH), September 2017. Available online. URL: www.nccih.nih.gov/health/mind-and-body-practices. Accessed September 10, 2024.

Mind-Body Exercises

- Spinal manipulation is typically safe for healthy children, but rare, serious complications have been reported.

Follow the Centers for Disease Control and Prevention's (CDC) vaccination recommendations to safeguard your child against vaccine-preventable diseases (www.cdc.gov/vaccines-children). Vaccinating children helps protect both their health and the health of the community.

It is important to talk with your child's health-care provider about any complementary health approach you are using or considering for your child. Encourage your teenagers to do the same.[2]

Section 30.2 | Yoga for Health and Wellness

WHAT IS YOGA, AND HOW DOES IT WORK?

Yoga is an ancient and complex practice rooted in Indian philosophy. It began as a spiritual practice but has become popular as a way of promoting physical and mental well-being. Although classical yoga includes other elements, yoga as practiced in the United States typically emphasizes physical postures (*asanas*), breathing techniques (*pranayama*), and meditation (*dyana*). Yoga, along with two practices of Chinese origin—tai chi and qigong—is sometimes called a "meditative movement" practice. All three include both meditative and physical elements. There are many styles of yoga, ranging from gentle practices to physically demanding ones. Differences in the types of yoga used in research studies may affect study results, making it challenging to evaluate the health effects of yoga.

HOW POPULAR IS YOGA IN THE UNITED STATES?

According to a national survey, the percentage of U.S. adults who practiced yoga increased from 5.0 percent in 2002 to 15.8 percent

---

[2] "Seven Things to Know about Mind and Body Practices for Children and Teens," National Center for Complementary and Integrative Health (NCCIH), April 2, 2017. Available online. URL: www.nccih.nih.gov/health/tips/things-to-know-about-mind-and-body-practices-for-children-and-teens. Accessed September 10, 2024.

in 2022. For children, 2017 data show that 8.4 percent of U.S. children aged 4–17 practiced yoga.

WHY DO AMERICANS PRACTICE YOGA?
A national survey data showed that 94 percent of adults who practiced yoga did it for wellness-related reasons, while 17.5 percent did it to treat a specific health condition. Some people reported doing both.

DO DIFFERENT GROUPS OF PEOPLE HAVE DIFFERENT EXPERIENCES WITH YOGA?
Much of the research on yoga in the United States has been conducted in predominantly female, non-Hispanic white, well-educated people with relatively high incomes. Other groups—particularly minority groups and those with lower incomes—have been underrepresented in yoga studies.

Different groups of people may have different yoga-related experiences, and the results of studies that did not examine a diverse population may not apply to everyone.

WHAT ARE THE HEALTH BENEFITS OF YOGA?
Research suggests that yoga may offer several benefits, including the following:
- Help improve general wellness by relieving stress, supporting good health habits, and improving mental/emotional health, sleep, and balance.
- Relieve neck pain, migraine or tension-type headaches, and pain associated with knee osteoarthritis. It may also have a small benefit for low-back pain.
- Help people with overweight or obesity lose weight.
- Help people quit smoking.
- Help people manage anxiety symptoms or depression.
- Relieve menopause symptoms.
- Be a helpful addition to treatment programs for substance use disorders.
- Help people with chronic diseases manage their symptoms and improve their quality of life (QOL).

Mind-Body Exercises

WHAT DOES RESEARCH SHOW ABOUT YOGA FOR WELLNESS?
Studies have suggested possible benefits of yoga for several aspects of wellness, including stress management, mental/emotional health, promoting healthy eating/activity habits, sleep, and balance.

CAN YOGA HELP WITH PAIN MANAGEMENT?
Yoga has been researched for several pain conditions, including low-back pain, neck pain, headaches, and knee osteoarthritis. Significant research has been done on low-back pain, and the evidence suggests a slight benefit. The evidence for other conditions looks promising, but the amount of research is relatively small.

IS PRACTICING YOGA A GOOD WAY TO LOSE WEIGHT?
There is evidence that yoga may help people lose weight.

IS YOGA HELPFUL FOR PEOPLE WITH CHRONIC DISEASES?
There is promising evidence that yoga may help people with some chronic diseases manage their symptoms and improve their QOL. Thus, yoga could be a helpful addition to treatment programs.

WHAT DOES RESEARCH SHOW ABOUT PRACTICING YOGA DURING PREGNANCY?
Physical activities such as yoga are safe and desirable for most pregnant women, as long as appropriate precautions are taken. Yoga may have health benefits for pregnant women, such as decreasing stress, anxiety, and depression.

DOES YOGA HAVE BENEFITS FOR CHILDREN?
Research suggests that yoga may have several potential benefits for children.

WHAT ARE THE RISKS OF YOGA?
Yoga is generally considered a safe form of physical activity for healthy people when performed properly under the guidance

of a qualified instructor. However, as with other forms of physical activity, injuries can occur. The most common injuries are sprains and strains, with the knee or lower leg being the most commonly injured parts. Serious injuries are rare. The risk of injury associated with yoga is lower than that for higher-impact physical activities.

Older adults may need to be particularly cautious when practicing yoga. The rate of yoga-related injuries treated in emergency departments is higher in people aged 65 and older than in younger adults.

To reduce your chances of getting hurt while doing yoga, consider the following precautions:

- Practice yoga under the guidance of a qualified instructor. Learning yoga on your own without supervision has been associated with increased risks.
- If you are new to yoga, avoid extreme practices such as headstands, shoulder stands, the lotus position, and forceful breathing.
- Be aware that hot yoga has special risks related to overheating and dehydration.
- Pregnant women, older adults, and people with health conditions should talk with their healthcare providers and the yoga instructor about their individual needs. They may need to avoid or modify some yoga poses and practices. Conditions that may require modifications include preexisting injuries (such as knee or hip injuries), lumbar spine disease, severe high blood pressure (HBP), balance issues, and glaucoma.[1]

---

[1] "Yoga: Effectiveness and Safety," National Center for Complementary and Integrative Health (NCCIH), August 2023. Available online. URL: www.nccih.nih.gov/health/yoga-effectiveness-and-safety. Accessed September 9, 2024.

Mind-Body Exercises

Section 30.3 | Tai Chi and Qigong

TAI CHI
What Is Tai Chi?
Tai chi is a practice that involves a series of slow, gentle movements and physical postures, a meditative state of mind, and controlled breathing. Tai chi originated as an ancient martial art in China. Over the years, it has become more focused on health promotion and rehabilitation.

Does Tai Chi Improve the Quality of Life of Older Adults?
A 2020 review of 13 studies (869 participants) found that tai chi had a small positive effect on the quality of life (QOL) and depressive symptoms of older adults with chronic conditions who lived in community settings. No significant effect was seen for mobility and physical endurance. The tai chi interventions involved 40- to 90-minute sessions done one to four times per week for 10–24 weeks. The authors said the studies had many differences among them, that the evidence was of low quality, and that larger, high-quality studies are needed.

Does Tai Chi Reduce Pain?
Some research suggests that tai chi may help reduce pain in people with low-back pain, fibromyalgia, and knee osteoarthritis. However, it is unclear whether tai chi is effective for alleviating pain from rheumatoid arthritis.

Is Tai Chi Safe during Pregnancy?
There are no published studies on the safety of tai chi during pregnancy. However, physical activities such as tai chi are likely safe and desirable during pregnancy in most instances, as long as appropriate precautions are taken. If you are pregnant, talk with your health-care providers before starting tai chi.

Tai chi during pregnancy may help with blood circulation, balance, coordination, strength, relaxation, and mental health, but research is needed in these areas.

Can Tai Chi Be Harmful?
Tai chi appears to be safe. A 2019 review of 24 studies (1,794 participants) found that the frequency of adverse events was similar for people doing tai chi, another active intervention, or no intervention. The review also found that in studies of people with heart failure, people in tai chi groups experienced fewer serious adverse events than people receiving no intervention. None of the serious adverse events reported in the 24 studies were thought to be caused by either tai chi or the control conditions (active interventions or no intervention). The adverse events that were reported as related to tai chi or other active interventions were minor, such as musculoskeletal aches and pain.

Tips to Consider
- Do not use tai chi to postpone seeing a health-care provider about a medical problem.
- Ask about the training and experience of the tai chi instructor you are considering.
- Take charge of your health. Talk with your health-care providers about any complementary health approaches you use. Together, you can make shared, well-informed decisions.[1]

QIGONG
What Is Qigong, and How Does It Work?
Qigong, pronounced "chi gong," was developed in China thousands of years ago as part of traditional Chinese medicine. It involves using exercises to optimize energy within the body, mind, and spirit, with the goal of improving and maintaining health and well-being. Qigong has both psychological and physical components and involves the regulation of the mind, breath, and body's movement and posture.

---

[1] "Tai Chi: What You Need to Know," National Center for Complementary and Integrative Health (NCCIH), December 2023. Available online. URL: www.nccih.nih.gov/health/tai-chi-what-you-need-to-know. Accessed September 10, 2024.

Mind-Body Exercises

In most forms of qigong:
- breath is slow, long, and deep; breath patterns may switch from abdominal breathing to breathing combined with speech sounds
- movements are typically gentle and smooth, aimed at relaxation
- mind regulation includes focusing one's attention and visualization

Dynamic (active) qigong techniques primarily focus on body movements, especially movements of the whole body or arms and legs. Meditative (passive) qigong techniques can be practiced in any posture that can be maintained over time and involve breath and mind exercises, with almost no body movement.

Is Qigong the Same as Tai Chi?
Tai chi originated as an ancient martial art, but over the years it has become more focused on health promotion and rehabilitation. When tai chi is performed for health, it is considered a form of qigong and involves integrated physical postures, focused attention, and controlled breathing. Tai chi is one of the hundreds of forms of qigong exercises that were developed in China. Other forms of qigong include Baduanjin, Liuzijue, Hu Yue Xian, Yijin Jing, and medical qigong.

Can Qigong Help Older Adults?
The number of studies examining qigong's effects on older adults is limited. Two reviews from 2019 explored qigong's influence on the physical and psychological health of older adults, with some positive findings.

Can Qigong Reduce Pain?
The research on qigong's role in pain reduction is mixed. Three reviews from 2018 to 2019, which included some studies, suggested that qigong may help decrease pain in community-dwelling older adults (160 participants), neck pain (525 participants), and

musculoskeletal pain in people aged 15–80 (1,787 participants). However, a 2020 review of five studies (576 participants) found conflicting results regarding qigong's effectiveness in reducing low-back and neck pain.

Is It Safe to Do Qigong during Pregnancy?

There is no research on the safety of qigong during pregnancy and extremely limited research on practicing qigong while pregnant. Pregnant women should talk with their health-care providers before starting qigong. Pregnant women may need to avoid or modify some qigong movements.

Can Qigong Be Harmful?

Qigong appears to be a safe form of activity. Many studies have indicated no negative side effects in people practicing qigong, including people with chronic diseases and older adults. A review of adults with neck pain included two studies that found that qigong and other exercise groups had similar side effects, which occurred in less than 10 percent of the adults and included muscle pain, soreness, and headache.

Tips to Consider

- Do not use qigong to postpone seeing a health-care provider about a medical problem.
- Ask about the training and experience of the qigong instructor you are considering.
- Take charge of your health. Talk with your health-care providers about any complementary health approaches you use. Together, you can make shared, well-informed decisions.[2]

---

[2] "Qigong: What You Need to Know," National Center for Complementary and Integrative Health (NCCIH), February 2022. Available online. URL: www.nccih.nih.gov/health/qigong-what-you-need-to-know. Accessed September 10, 2024.

Mind-Body Exercises

Section 30.4 | **Meditation and Mindfulness**

WHAT ARE MEDITATION AND MINDFULNESS?

Meditation has a history that goes back thousands of years, and many meditative techniques began in Eastern traditions. The term "meditation" refers to a variety of practices that focus on mind and body integration and are used to calm the mind and enhance overall well-being. Some types of meditation involve maintaining mental focus on a particular sensation, such as breathing, a sound, a visual image, or a mantra, which is a repeated word or phrase. Other forms of meditation include the practice of mindfulness, which involves maintaining attention or awareness of the present moment without making judgments.

Programs that teach meditation or mindfulness may combine these practices with other activities. For example, mindfulness-based stress reduction teaches mindful meditation, but it also includes discussion sessions and other strategies to help people apply what they have learned to stressful experiences. Mindfulness-based cognitive therapy integrates mindfulness practices with aspects of cognitive behavioral therapy.

WHY DO PEOPLE PRACTICE MINDFULNESS MEDITATION?

In a 2012 U.S. survey, 1.9 percent of 34,525 adults reported that they had practiced mindfulness meditation in the past 12 months. Among those respondents who practiced mindfulness meditation exclusively, 73 percent reported that they meditated for their general wellness and to prevent diseases, and most of them (approximately 92 percent) reported that they meditated to relax or reduce stress. In more than half of the responses, a desire for better sleep was a reason for practicing mindfulness meditation.

HOW POPULAR ARE MEDITATION AND MINDFULNESS?

According to the National Health Interview Survey, an annual nationally representative survey, the percentage of U.S. adults who practiced meditation more than doubled between 2002 and 2022, from 7.5 to 17.3 percent. Of seven complementary health approaches for which data were collected in the 2022 survey, meditation was the most popular, surpassing yoga (used by 15.8 percent of adults), chiropractic care (11.0 percent), massage therapy (10.9 percent), guided imagery/progressive muscle relaxation (6.4 percent), acupuncture (2.2 percent), and naturopathy (1.3 percent).

For children aged 4–17 years, data are available for 2017; in that year, 5.4 percent of U.S. children practiced meditation.

WHAT ARE THE HEALTH BENEFITS OF MEDITATION AND MINDFULNESS?

Meditation and mindfulness practices may have a variety of health benefits and may help people improve the quality of their lives. Recent studies have investigated if meditation or mindfulness helps people manage anxiety, stress, depression, pain, or symptoms related to withdrawal from nicotine, alcohol, or opioids.

Other studies have looked at the effects of meditation or mindfulness on weight control or sleep quality.

However, much of the research on these topics has been preliminary or not scientifically rigorous. Because the studies examined many types of meditation and mindfulness practices and the effects of those practices are hard to measure, the results have been difficult to analyze and may have been interpreted too optimistically.

HOW DO MEDITATION AND MINDFULNESS WORK?

Some research suggests that meditation and mindfulness practices may affect the functioning or structure of the brain. Studies have used various methods of measuring brain activity to look for measurable differences in the brains of people engaged in mindfulness-based practices. Other studies have theorized that training in meditation and mindfulness practices can change brain activity. However, the results of these studies are difficult to interpret, and the practical implications are not clear.

ARE MEDITATION AND MINDFULNESS PRACTICES SAFE?

Meditation and mindfulness practices usually are considered to have few risks. However, few studies have examined these practices

Mind-Body Exercises

for potentially harmful effects, so it is not possible to make definite statements about safety.

TIPS TO CONSIDER
- Do not use meditation or mindfulness to replace conventional care or as a reason to postpone seeing a health-care provider about a medical problem.
- Ask about the training and experience of the instructor of the meditation or mindfulness practice you are considering.
- Take charge of your health—talk with your health-care providers about any complementary health approaches you use. Together, you can make shared, well-informed decisions.[1]

---

[1] "Meditation and Mindfulness: Effectiveness and Safety," National Center for Complementary and Integrative Health (NCCIH), June 1, 2022. Available online. URL: www.nccih.nih.gov/health/meditation-and-mindfulness-what-you-need-to-know. Accessed September 10, 2024.

Part 5 | Fitness Safety

Chapter 31 | Workout Safety

Chapter Contents
Section 31.1—The Essentials of Warming Up and
  Cooling Down 249
Section 31.2—Common Workout Mistakes and How to
  Avoid Them..252
Section 31.3—Physical Activity and Proper Gear......................254

Chapter 21
Workout Safety

Section 31.1 | The Essentials of Warming Up and Cooling Down

WHY WARM UP AND COOL DOWN
Warming up and cooling down can help prevent injury and reduce muscle soreness during physical activity, contributing to overall safety.
- Warming up prepares the muscles and heart for activity.
- Cooling down gradually slows the heart rate and helps prepare the muscles for future activity.

WHAT IS IN A WARM-UP?
Warming up prepares the body for activity, and helps prevent injury and reduce muscle soreness.
    A warm-up may take 5–15 minutes:
- Perform the planned activity, such as walking, at a lower intensity (slower pace) for a brief time. This could mean walking slowly for a few minutes before increasing speed.
- If planning to do something more vigorous than walking, perform a few minutes of gentle stretching after the warm-up.

ENGAGE THE CORE
The body's core muscles include those around the trunk, pelvis (hips), and back. This is where the center of gravity is located. All body movements involve the core muscles, and awareness of core muscles is important during physical activity.
- Weak core muscles can lead to poor posture, back pain, and a higher risk of injury.
- Strong core muscles improve posture, balance, and movement and support the back.

INCREASE CARDIOVASCULAR ACTIVITY
Cardiovascular activity involves large muscles moving rhythmically for a sustained period. It causes the heart to beat faster. Examples

include brisk walking, running, bicycling, jumping rope, and swimming.

Cardiovascular activity has three components:
1. **Intensity**. How hard the body works during the activity. Intensity can be moderate (e.g., brisk walking) or vigorous (e.g., running or jogging).
2. **Frequency**. How often cardiovascular activity is performed.
3. **Duration**. How long each session lasts.

INCREASE DAILY STEPS

Walking is an excellent way to stay physically active. It is free, enjoyable, and can be done almost anywhere. Walking daily is more beneficial than occasional weekend activities. Consider using a pedometer or fitness tracker to measure steps and challenge yourself to increase your daily count.

Six reasons to get up and walk:
1. Brisk walking has many health benefits.
2. Walking burns calories, which, combined with a healthy diet, helps manage weight.
3. More than half of the body's muscles are designed for walking, making it a natural movement.
4. Brisk walking is a cardiovascular activity that strengthens the heart, lungs, and muscles.
5. Walking refreshes the mind, reduces fatigue, increases energy, and improves sleep.
6. Walking can be a fun way to socialize with friends and family.

INCREASE STRENGTH TRAINING

Strength training improves endurance, muscle and bone strength, coordination, and balance. It can be done with or without equipment. To increase resistance and intensity, use body weight, free weights, resistance bands, or resistance tubes.

Six reasons to do strength training:
1. Helps the body burn more calories.
2. Stronger muscles reduce stress on the joints.

Workout Safety

3. Prevents muscle loss associated with aging.
4. Makes household chores and daily activities easier.
5. Improves the body's ability to use insulin and maintain healthy blood sugar levels.
6. Protects independence as you age and reduces the likelihood of falls.

INCREASE FLEXIBILITY

Stretching increases the range of motion, making it easier to perform daily tasks and enjoy recreational activities. Always warm up with light activity before stretching. Stretching after strength or cardiovascular activities is also beneficial. Aim to stretch every day. If that is not possible, try to stretch at least three times a week for 20 minutes per session.

WHAT IS IN A COOLDOWN?

Cooling down after physical activity helps prevent injury and reduces muscle soreness. It gradually slows the heart rate and prepares the muscles for the next workout.

A cooldown may take 5–15 minutes:
- To cool down, continue the activity but slow the pace to lower the heart rate.
- Stretch all major muscle groups used during the activity. Stretching muscles while they are warm helps increase flexibility.

Warming up and cooling down are essential components of any workout routine, helping prevent injury and improve muscle recovery, which contributes to overall safety. Incorporating strength, flexibility, and cardiovascular activities into a regular fitness routine enhances overall physical health, allowing for continued physical activity and well-being.[1]

---

[1] "Pump Up Your Physical Activity," U.S. Department of Veterans Affairs (VA), June 27, 2019. Available online. URL: www.move.va.gov/docs/veteranworkbook/movewbm09.pdf. Accessed September 8, 2024.

Section 31.2 | Common Workout Mistakes and How to Avoid Them

Finding or making time to exercise is the first step toward improving your health, but it is not the only step. Workouts can be challenging, and mistakes in the gym are common. These mistakes can sometimes cause mild strains or even significant injuries. By making small adjustments to your routine, you can begin to see incredible results.

THE ALL-OR-NOTHING APPROACH
Not having a full hour to exercise is no reason to skip your workout. Research shows that even 10 minutes of exercise can provide important health benefits.

UNBALANCED STRENGTH-TRAINING PROGRAMS
Many people focus on certain muscles, such as the abdominals or biceps, because they have a greater effect on appearance or are where they feel strongest. To achieve a strong, balanced body, you need to train all major muscle groups.

BAD FORM
The surest way to get injured in a gym is to use improper form. For example, allowing the knee to extend beyond the toes during a lunge or squat can put undue stress on the knee, and using momentum to lift heavy weights or not exercising through a full range of motion will result in less-than-optimal outcomes.

NOT PROGRESSING WISELY
Exercising too much, too hard, or too often is a common mistake. Rest and gradual progression are important components of a safe and effective exercise program.

NOT ENOUGH VARIETY
Many people find a routine or activity they enjoy and never change it. Unchanging workouts can lead to boredom, plateaus, and, in the worst case, injury or burnout.

NOT ADJUSTING MACHINES TO FIT YOUR BODY SIZE
Most exercise equipment is designed to accommodate a wide range of body types. However, it is important to adjust each machine to your unique needs. Using improperly adjusted machines can result in suboptimal outcomes and increase your risk of injury.

FOCUSING ON ANYTHING BUT YOUR WORKOUT
It is crucial to be mindful of your workout. Distractions, such as reading or watching TV, can adversely affect the quality of your workout by slowing you down.

SKIPPING THE COOL DOWN
Too many people finish their workout and head straight to the showers. Taking a few minutes to cool down, lower their heart rate, and stretch their muscles is important for flexibility and preparing their bodies for the next workout.

POOR GYM ETIQUETTE
Poor etiquette can include lingering on machines long after you are done, chatting loudly on your phone, or neglecting to wipe your sweat from equipment. Always be considerate of others.

NOT SETTING REALISTIC GOALS
Unrealistic or vague goals are among the leading causes of exercise dropout. Set specific, achievable goals that challenge you without being overly difficult.[1]

---

[1] Brookhaven National Laboratory (BNL), "American Council on Exercise (ACE's) Top Ten Mistakes People Make in the Gym," U.S. Department of Energy (DOE), January 23, 2007. Available online. URL: www.bnl.gov/bera/docs/pdf/exercise-ace.pdf. Accessed September 10, 2024.

Section 31.3 | **Physical Activity and Proper Gear**

WHY PHYSICAL ACTIVITY IS IMPORTANT
You may wonder if being physically active is really worth the time and effort. Many people think so! They know that being active is a great way to have fun and spend time with friends. Fitness can also do amazing things for both the mind and body.

HOW PHYSICAL ACTIVITY BENEFITS MENTAL HEALTH
Did you know that being physically active can improve how you feel? It can also help you perform better in tasks and even improve your mood and behavior. This is partly because physical activity triggers the release of "feel-good" chemicals called "endorphins." Regular physical activity may help by:
- reducing stress
- improving sleep
- boosting energy levels
- reducing symptoms of anxiety and depression
- increasing self-esteem
- making you feel proud for taking care of yourself
- enhancing overall performance in daily tasks

HOW PHYSICAL ACTIVITY BENEFITS THE BODY
Being physically active is great for the muscles, heart, and lungs. Some additional benefits of regular physical activity include:
- **Building strong bones**. The body creates the most bone mass during childhood and adolescence.
- **Promoting a healthy weight**. Obesity is a serious problem among people in the United States. It can cause sleep problems, joint issues, heart problems, emotional difficulties, and more, but exercise can help.
- **Helping prevent diabetes**. An increasing number of people are being diagnosed with diabetes. Regular physical activity can help prevent type 2 diabetes.

Workout Safety

- **Building healthy habits.** If you get into the habit of being active now, you are more likely to continue being active as you grow older.
- **Fighting cancer.** Research suggests that exercise may help protect against certain types of cancer.
- **Helping prevent high blood pressure (HBP).** The number of people with HBP is growing. HBP makes the heart and arteries work harder, increasing the risk of kidney and eye disease.

WHAT TO WEAR DURING A WORKOUT

Are you wondering what to wear when working out? Many activities do not require special clothing, but in some cases, clothing choices do matter. Anyone who is working out looks cool, regardless of their outfit!

HOW TO CHOOSE WORKOUT CLOTHES

When selecting workout clothes, consider the following:
- **Avoid tight clothing.** You need to move freely. Wearing loose clothing also allows air to reach your skin and dry sweat, keeping you cool.
- **Choose the right colors.** In the summer, lighter colors help keep you cool, while darker clothes help trap heat and keep you warm in winter.
- **Wear layers in cold weather.** You can remove layers as you warm up.
- **Protect your head.** Wear a hat or cap for sun protection, and in cold weather, choose a wool or ski cap to stay warm.
- **Choose the right fabric.** If you expect to sweat, choose fabrics that wick moisture away from your skin. Try synthetics like polypropylene. Cotton may be less comfortable because it holds moisture longer.

Fitness and Exercise Sourcebook, Seventh Edition

HOW TO PICK THE RIGHT WORKOUT SHOES

Wearing the right shoes when working out is essential. Follow these tips to find the best pair:

- **Protect your feet**. Choose shoes that are sturdy and have cushioned soles. They should also provide arch support.
- **Choose shoes for the activity**. If you plan to run or play a specific sport often, choose shoes made for that activity. For example, tennis players should wear tennis shoes, and runners should wear running shoes. Ask a sports shoe salesperson for advice.
- **Get the right fit**. Ask a salesperson to measure your foot and check the fit. The wrong fit can lead to discomfort or even foot problems. Try shopping at the end of the day when your feet are slightly larger, just as they are when you exercise. Also, try on shoes with the socks you plan to wear during workouts.

HOW TO PICK THE RIGHT EQUIPMENT

The right equipment, from helmets to shoes, can help keep you safe during sports or physical activities.

- **Helmets**. Helmets protect you from head injuries when there is a risk of falling or being hit in the head, such as in baseball, biking, skiing, horseback riding, skateboarding, and inline skating. Make sure the helmet is designed for the specific activity and fits correctly. In some states, wearing a helmet while biking is required by law. Bike helmets should have a sticker from the U.S. Consumer Product Safety Commission (CPSC).
- **Special eye protection**. Eye protection helps prevent sports-related eye injuries in activities such as basketball, baseball, hockey, and racquet sports. Regular glasses or sunglasses will not protect against injuries. If you wear regular glasses, protective eyewear should fit over them. Goggles made from polycarbonate are extremely strong and should fit snugly with cushioning. Ask a coach or eye doctor about appropriate eye protection.

Workout Safety

- **Mouth guards**. Mouth guards protect the mouth, teeth, and tongue in sports such as soccer, lacrosse, basketball, baseball, and more. Mouth guards are available at sporting goods stores or from your dentist.
- **Pads for wrists, knees, and elbows**. Pads help prevent injuries, including broken bones, during activities such as inline skating, snowboarding, and hockey. In some sports, such as soccer, shin guards may be required by your coach to protect the lower legs.
- **Shoes**. Shoes should fit well and be appropriate for the sport. Consult your coach or an athletic shoe salesperson for guidance, and ask how often shoes need to be replaced.

Physical activity offers numerous benefits for both mental and physical health, from reducing stress to preventing serious health conditions. By wearing the right clothing, shoes, and safety equipment, you can enjoy physical activities while staying safe and comfortable.[1]

---

[1] girlshealth.gov, "Safety Equipment," Office on Women's Health (OWH), July 1, 2015. Available online. URL: www.girlshealth.gov/fitness/fitnesssafety/equipment.html. Accessed September 10, 2024.

Chapter 32 | Nutrition and Exercise

Chapter Contents
Section 32.1—Hydration and Health..261
Section 32.2—Nutrition for an Active Lifestyle 263
Section 32.3—Dietary Supplements for Exercise......................266
Section 32.4—Anabolic Steroids and Other Performance-
 Enhancing Drugs 269
Section 32.5—The Risks of Bodybuilding Products
 Containing Steroids 274

Section 32.1 | **Hydration and Health**

BENEFITS OF DRINKING WATER

Getting enough water each day is essential for maintaining good health and supporting exercise. Drinking water prevents dehydration, which can lead to unclear thinking, mood changes, overheating, constipation, and kidney stones. Water contains no calories, so replacing sugary drinks with plain water can help reduce caloric intake.

Water helps the body by:
- keeping a normal temperature, which is especially important during exercise
- lubricating and cushioning joints
- protecting the spinal cord and other sensitive tissues
- eliminating waste through urination, perspiration, and bowel movements

WHEN YOUR BODY NEEDS MORE WATER

Your body requires more water when you are:
- in hot climates
- more physically active or exercising
- running a fever
- experiencing diarrhea or vomiting

MEETING DAILY WATER INTAKE

Daily water intake recommendations vary by age, sex, activity level, pregnancy status, and breastfeeding status. Most water intake comes from drinking water and other beverages, but foods with high water content, such as many fruits and vegetables, also contribute to fluid intake.

TIPS TO DRINK MORE WATER

- Carry a reusable water bottle with you, especially during exercise.
- Freeze water in freezer-safe bottles for ice-cold water throughout the day.

- Choose water over sugary drinks.
- Opt for water when eating out.
- Serve water during meals.
- Add a wedge of lime or lemon to your water for flavor.

HEALTHIER DRINK OPTIONS
Many beverages can be part of a healthy eating pattern:
- **Low- or no-calorie beverages.** Plain coffee or tea, sparkling water, seltzer, and flavored water are low-calorie options.
- **Drinks with important nutrients.** Low-fat or fat-free milk, unsweetened fortified milk alternatives, and 100 percent fruit or vegetable juice contain important nutrients. These should be consumed within the recommended calorie limits.

Other Beverages
- **Sugary drinks.** Regular sodas, fruit drinks, sports drinks, energy drinks, sweetened waters, and sweetened coffee or tea contain calories but little nutritional value.
- **Alcoholic drinks.** If you choose to drink alcohol, do so in moderation.
- **Caffeinated drinks.** Moderate caffeine consumption (up to 400 mg per day) can be part of a healthy diet. This is about 3–5 cups of plain coffee.
- **Drinks with sugar alternatives.** Drinks labeled as "sugar-free" or "diet" often contain high-intensity sweeteners such as sucralose, aspartame, or saccharine. While these sweeteners may reduce caloric intake in the short term, questions remain about their long-term effectiveness for weight management.
- **Energy drinks.** In addition to added sugar, energy drinks may contain large amounts of caffeine and other legal stimulants. There are concerns about the potential health risks of these products, particularly for young people.[1]

---

[1] "About Water and Healthier Drinks," Centers for Disease Control and Prevention (CDC), January 2, 2024. Available online. URL: www.cdc.gov/healthy-weight-growth/water-healthy-drinks. Accessed September 11, 2024.

Nutrition and Exercise

TIPS FOR STAYING HYDRATED
- Drink when you feel thirsty, or even before.
- Drink water before, during, and after exercise.
- Choose water or other low-calorie beverages, such as plain coffee, tea, or sparkling water.
- Carry a water bottle and refill it as needed throughout the day.
- Drink at regular intervals, such as with meals.
- Consume extra fluids in hot weather or when feeling unwell.

Seek medical attention immediately if you experience confusion, fainting, a rapid heartbeat or breathing, or an inability to urinate.[2]

Section 32.2 | Nutrition for an Active Lifestyle

Eating healthy means following a balanced eating pattern that includes a variety of nutritious foods and drinks. It also involves consuming the right number of calories for your needs, while avoiding both over- and under-eating.

CHOOSE A MIX OF HEALTHY FOODS
There are plenty of healthy options in every food group. Choose a variety of foods you enjoy, including:
- whole fruits such as apples, berries, oranges, mango, and bananas
- vegetables such as broccoli, sweet potatoes, beets, okra, spinach, peppers, and jicama
- whole grains such as brown rice, millet, oatmeal, bulgur, and whole-wheat bread
- proteins such as lean meats, chicken, eggs, seafood, beans, lentils, nuts, seeds, and tofu

---

[2] *NIH News in Health*, "Hydrating for Health," National Institutes of Health (NIH), May 2023. Available online. URL: https://newsinhealth.nih.gov/2023/05/hydrating-health. Accessed September 10, 2024.

- low-fat or fat-free dairy such as milk, yogurt, cheese, lactose-free dairy, and fortified soy beverages or soy yogurt
- oils such as vegetable oil, olive oil, and oils found in foods including seafood, avocado, and nuts

LIMIT CERTAIN NUTRIENTS AND INGREDIENTS
- **Sodium (salt).** Table salt contains sodium, but most of the sodium we consume comes from packaged foods or restaurant meals.
- **Added sugars.** These include syrups and sweeteners that manufacturers add to products such as sodas, yogurt, and cereals—as well as sugars you add yourself, such as in coffee.
- **Saturated fat.** This comes from animal products such as cheese, fatty meats, poultry, whole milk, butter, and many sweets. Certain plant products, such as palm and coconut oils, also contain saturated fats.

HEALTH BENEFITS
A healthy eating routine can significantly contribute to your overall well-being. Making smart food choices can help you manage your weight and reduce the risk of chronic diseases such as:
- overweight and obesity
- heart disease
- type 2 diabetes
- high blood pressure (HBP)
- certain types of cancer

TAKE ACTION: MAKE SMALL CHANGES
Making small adjustments to your eating habits can have a lasting positive effect on your health. Make healthy swaps. Start by making one or two small changes each week, such as:
- Drink sparkling water instead of soda.
- Try plain, low-fat yogurt with fruit instead of full-fat yogurt with added sugars.

Nutrition and Exercise

- Choose low-sodium black beans instead of regular canned black beans.
- Cook with olive oil instead of butter.

SHOP SMART
Plan ahead for healthy grocery shopping:
- Make a shopping list and stick to it.
- Do not shop when you are hungry; eat something before going to the store.

Use these tips to make healthy choices:
- Try a variety of colorful vegetables and fruits.
- Choose fat-free or low-fat dairy products, or opt for soy milk and soy yogurt with added calcium, vitamin A, and vitamin D.
- Opt for lower-calorie, lower-sodium, and lower-sugar options.
- Choose foods made with whole grains such as whole-wheat bread, cereal, and pasta.
- Buy lean cuts of meat and poultry, and incorporate more plant-based proteins such as fish, shellfish, beans, and nuts.
- Save money by purchasing fruits and vegetables that are in season or on sale.

CHECK THE LABEL
Reading the Nutrition Facts label helps you make informed choices. Start by looking at the serving size and the number of servings per package. Then, review the calorie count and balance it with your energy needs. Look at the percent Daily Value (% DV) to see if a food is higher or lower in specific nutrients. Choose foods that are:
- Low in added sugars, sodium, and saturated fat (5% DV or less).
- High in fiber, calcium, potassium, iron, and vitamin D (20% DV or more).

HEALTHY FAMILIES

Parents and caregivers can model healthy eating habits for children by teaching them how to select and prepare nutritious snacks and meals. You can still eat healthy while away from home. Consider these tips:

- Pack snacks such as fruit, unsalted nuts, or low-fat string cheese.
- Check for calorie information on restaurant menus.
- Choose dishes that are steamed, baked, or grilled instead of fried.
- Ask for meals to be prepared without added salt.

SEE YOUR DOCTOR

If you are concerned about your eating habits, talk to your doctor. A doctor may refer you to a registered dietitian, a professional who can provide personalized guidance on healthy eating.

Making smart food choices and eating a variety of nutritious foods can improve your overall health and help manage your weight. By making small changes over time, you can significantly reduce your risk for chronic diseases and enjoy the long-term benefits of a healthy lifestyle.[1]

Section 32.3 | Dietary Supplements for Exercise

THE ROLE OF DIET AND SUPPLEMENTS

If you regularly exercise—or especially if you compete in sports—you know that a nutritionally adequate diet and proper hydration are essential for maximizing physical performance. However, you might wonder if dietary supplements could help you train harder, improve performance, or gain a competitive edge.

---

[1] Office of Disease Prevention and Health Promotion (ODPHP), "Eat Healthy," U.S. Department of Health and Human Services (HHS), July 14, 2022. Available online. URL: https://health.gov/myhealthfinder/health-conditions/diabetes/eat-healthy. Accessed September 10, 2024.

Nutrition and Exercise

Performance supplements cannot replace a healthy diet, but some may offer benefits depending on the type and intensity of your activity. Others may be ineffective, and a few could even be harmful.

Before considering a performance supplement, consult your health-care provider. If you have a coach or trainer knowledgeable about sports medicine, ask them as well. This is particularly important if you are a teenager or have medical conditions. It is also essential to know whether the medications you take could interact with any supplements.

INGREDIENTS IN SUPPLEMENTS

Performance supplements often contain a variety of ingredients—such as vitamins, minerals, protein, amino acids, and herbs—in varying amounts and combinations. They come in many forms, including capsules, tablets, liquids, and powders.

It is worth noting that manufacturers of performance supplements typically do not conduct extensive studies to verify the safety and efficacy of their products. When research is done, it usually involves small groups of young, healthy men for short periods. Research may not include women, older adults, or teenagers, and it may not apply to your specific athletic activity.

Common Ingredients in Supplements
- antioxidants (vitamin C, vitamin E, and coenzyme Q_{10})
- arginine
- beetroot or beet juice
- beta-alanine
- beta-hydroxy-beta-methylbutyrate (HMB)
- betaine
- branched-chain amino acids (BCAAs)
- caffeine
- citrulline
- creatine
- deer antler velvet
- dehydroepiandrosterone (DHEA)
- ginseng

- glutamine
- iron
- protein
- quercetin
- ribose
- sodium bicarbonate
- tart or sour cherry
- *Tribulus terrestris*

REGULATION OF PERFORMANCE SUPPLEMENTS

The U.S. Food and Drug Administration (FDA) regulates dietary supplements differently from prescription or over-the-counter (OTC) drugs. The FDA does not test or approve performance supplements before they are marketed. Manufacturers are responsible for ensuring the safety of their supplements and the accuracy of their product labels.

If the FDA finds an unsafe dietary supplement, it can remove the product from the market or request a recall. The FDA and the Federal Trade Commission (FTC) can also take action against companies making false claims, adding pharmaceutical drugs or illegal substances to their products, or promoting supplements as treatments for diseases.

CAN DIETARY SUPPLEMENTS FOR EXERCISE AND ATHLETIC PERFORMANCE BE HARMFUL?

As with all dietary supplements, performance supplements may cause side effects and interact with prescription or OTC medications. Many of these products contain multiple ingredients that have not been sufficiently tested in combination.

Interactions with Medications

Certain supplements can interact with medications. For example, ginseng may reduce the blood-thinning effects of warfarin (Coumadin), and cimetidine (Tagamet HB) can slow caffeine metabolism, increasing the risk of side effects. Always inform your health-care provider if you are using supplements alongside medications.

Fraudulent and Adulterated Products

Some dietary supplements marketed for performance enhancement may contain undeclared or illegal ingredients, including stimulants, steroids, or prescription medications. The FDA has banned substances such as androstenedione, dimethylamylamine (DMAA), and ephedra due to safety concerns.

CHOOSING A SENSIBLE APPROACH TO IMPROVING EXERCISE AND ATHLETIC PERFORMANCE

If you are an athlete—whether competitive or recreational—you will perform best with a balanced diet, proper hydration, physical fitness, and appropriate training. While a few supplements have scientific backing for improving performance, athletes should only use them alongside proper diet and training, and under the guidance of health-care providers or sports-medicine professionals.

Most performance supplements should only be used by adults. The American Academy of Pediatrics advises that performance supplements do not enhance the abilities of teenage athletes beyond what proper nutrition and training can provide.[1]

Section 32.4 | Anabolic Steroids and Other Performance-Enhancing Drugs

WHAT ARE ANABOLIC STEROIDS AND OTHER APPEARANCE- AND PERFORMANCE-ENHANCING DRUGS?

Anabolic-androgenic steroids, often shortened to "anabolic steroids," "steroids," or "androgens," are the most widely misused APEDs. These synthetic substances are similar to the male sex hormone testosterone. They promote the growth of skeletal muscle (anabolic effects) and the development of male sexual characteristics (androgenic effects) in both males and females.

---

[1] Office of Dietary Supplements (ODS), "Dietary Supplements for Exercise and Athletic Performance," National Institutes of Health (NIH), March 22, 2021. Available online. URL: https://ods.od.nih.gov/factsheets/ExerciseAndAthleticPerformance-Consumer. Accessed September 10, 2024.

These compounds are sometimes used medically to treat delayed puberty and muscle loss due to disease, and to treat low levels of testosterone in men with an associated medical condition. Anabolic-androgenic steroids can also improve feelings of well-being and increase bone strength, but they are not approved for these purposes. However, testosterone-supplementation therapy is an increasingly common treatment for mood and sexual performance problems associated with male aging and is controversially being prescribed even for younger men.

Nonsteroidal anabolics include insulin, insulin-like growth factor (IGF), and human growth hormone (HGH)—substances that are produced by the human body and are prescribed for legitimate medical uses but are sometimes misused for performance enhancement.

Ergo/thermogenics are compounds used to decrease body fat or promote leanness versus muscle mass in endurance athletes. The three main categories of ergo/thermogenics are:

- **Xanthines**. Compounds that increase attention and wakefulness and suppress appetite. Examples include caffeine, the asthma drug theophylline, and theobromine—a substance found in chocolate, coffee, and tea.
- **Sympathomimetics**. Drugs similar in structure and action to epinephrine and norepinephrine—natural chemicals in the body that increase heart rate, constrict blood vessels, and raise blood pressure. An example is ephedrine, derived from the ephedra plant. Ephedrine/ephedra was previously included in dietary supplements that promoted weight loss, increased energy, and enhanced athletic performance.
- **Thyroid hormones**. Substances that regulate metabolism by altering the function of the thyroid. Cytomel is an example.

WHY ARE ANABOLIC STEROIDS MISUSED?

Anabolic steroids increase lean muscle mass when used in conjunction with weight training. For nonathlete weightlifters, the

Nutrition and Exercise

typical aim is the improvement of appearance. Steroid use is often associated with a form of male body dysmorphic disorder called "muscle dysmorphia," a preoccupation with the perceived inadequate size of one's muscles.

As a result, some users report taking anabolic steroids to increase confidence and because they feel they can no longer get bigger through weight training alone. Most users report that anabolic steroids help them achieve their ideal body.

Increasing muscle mass may also promote strength, which can improve performance in certain types of sports. Strength-dependent sports (e.g., weightlifting, shot put, football) receive more benefits than sports that require speed, agility, flexibility, and/or endurance.

Anabolic steroid users also report that their muscles recover faster from intense strain and muscle injury. Research in animals has not conclusively supported this belief, with some studies showing that anabolic steroids can enhance recovery from certain types of muscle damage, while others find no benefit in taking anabolic steroids to enhance muscle recovery.

Anabolic steroid users report using an average of about 11 APEDs per year. They are also more likely than nonsteroid users to take supplements such as protein powders and creatine; estrogen blockers; ergo/thermogenics, such as caffeine or ephedrine; medications for erectile dysfunction; and other hormones such as insulin, thyroid hormones, and human growth hormone.

COMMONLY MISUSED STEROIDS
Oral Steroids
- Anadrol (oxymetholone)
- Anavar (oxandrolone)
- Dianabol (methandienone)
- Winstrol (stanozolol)
- Restandol (testosterone undecanoate)

Injectable Steroids
- Deca-Durabolin (nandrolone decanoate)
- Durabolin (nandrolone phenpropionate)

- Depo-Testosterone (testosterone cypionate)
- Agovirin (testosterone propionate)
- Retandrol (testosterone phenylpropionate)
- Equipoise (boldenone undecylenate)

WHAT ARE THE SIDE EFFECTS OF ANABOLIC STEROID MISUSE?

A variety of side effects can occur when anabolic steroids are misused, ranging from mild effects to those that are harmful or even life-threatening. Most side effects are reversible if the user stops taking the drugs. However, some may be permanent or semi-permanent.

Most data on the long-term effects of anabolic steroids in humans come from case reports rather than formal epidemiological studies. Serious and life-threatening adverse effects may be underreported, especially since they may occur many years later. One review found 19 deaths in published case reports related to anabolic steroid use between 1990 and 2012; however, many steroid users also used other drugs, making it difficult to attribute these deaths solely to anabolic steroid use. One animal study found that exposing male mice for one fifth of their lifespan to steroid doses comparable to those taken by human athletes caused a high frequency of early deaths.

WHAT TREATMENTS ARE EFFECTIVE FOR ANABOLIC STEROID MISUSE?

People who use steroids often do not seek treatment for their use, with one study reporting that 56 percent of users had never informed their physician about their use. This may be because users feel their physician lacks knowledge about anabolic steroids. Additionally, many Internet sites devoted to anabolic steroids and other APEDs challenge the professionalism of health-care providers and offer their own medically questionable advice on the use of APEDs. This underscores the importance of health-care providers being educated on the signs and symptoms of steroid use in their patients.

Nutrition and Exercise

Current views recommend that treatment for steroid use address the underlying causes of steroid use. This can include:
- psychological therapies (and possibly medications) for muscle dysmorphia
- endocrine therapies to restore function in those suffering from hypogonadism and to alleviate symptoms of depression
- antidepressants for those whose depression does not respond to endocrine therapies
- pharmacological and psychosocial treatments for patients who are also dependent on opioids, which appear to be effective in alleviating signs of anabolic steroid dependence

WHAT CAN BE DONE TO PREVENT STEROID MISUSE?

Research suggests that high school athletes are less likely to use steroids if their peers and parents disapprove, indicating that peers and parents can be strong partners in prevention efforts.

However, research shows that simply teaching students about steroids' adverse effects does not convince adolescents that they will be adversely affected, nor does such instruction discourage young people from taking steroids in the future. Presenting both the risks and benefits of anabolic steroid use is more effective in convincing adolescents about steroids' negative effects, apparently because students find a balanced approach more credible.

Research also indicates that some adolescents misuse steroids as part of a pattern of high-risk behaviors, such as drinking and driving, carrying a gun, driving a motorcycle without a helmet, and using other illicit drugs. This suggests that a prevention program should focus on comprehensive high-risk behavior screening and counseling among teens who use anabolic steroids.[1]

---

[1] "Anabolic Steroids and Other Appearance and Performance Enhancing Drugs (APEDs)," National Institute on Drug Abuse (NIDA), May 2023. Available online. URL: https://nida.nih.gov/research-topics/anabolic-steroids. Accessed September 10, 2024.

Section 32.5 | The Risks of Bodybuilding Products Containing Steroids

BODYBUILDING PRODUCTS CAN BE RISKY

The U.S. Food and Drug Administration (FDA) has found that some bodybuilding products may illegally contain steroids or steroid-like substances associated with potentially serious health risks, including life-threatening liver injury. The FDA has received hundreds of adverse event reports, some of which include evidence of serious liver damage.

In addition to liver injury, anabolic steroids have been linked to severe reactions such as:
- severe acne
- hair loss
- altered mood
- irritability
- increased aggression
- depression

They have also been connected to life-threatening conditions, including:
- kidney damage
- heart attack
- stroke
- pulmonary embolism (blood clots in the lungs)
- deep vein thrombosis (blood clots in deep veins)

These bodybuilding products are often marketed as hormone products or as alternatives to anabolic steroids for increasing muscle mass and strength. Many claim to affect androgen, estrogen, or progestin-like activity in the body, but they may contain anabolic steroids or steroid-like substances, which are synthetic hormones related to testosterone.

BODYBUILDING PRODUCTS MAY CONTAIN STEROIDS

The FDA found that many of these bodybuilding products, labeled as "dietary supplements," are sold both online and in retail stores.

Nutrition and Exercise

However, many of these products are not true dietary supplements. Instead, they contain undisclosed or unproven ingredients and are illegally marketed as unapproved new drugs. The FDA has not reviewed these products for safety, effectiveness, or quality before they were marketed.

These potentially harmful and sometimes hidden ingredients in bodybuilding products continue to raise concerns. The companies producing and selling these products are breaking the law by exploiting accessible marketplaces, placing consumers at risk without fully understanding the dangers. Many of these products are promoted with claims of miraculous results or empty promises, misleading consumers.

Some individuals use bodybuilding products in combination, a practice called "stacking," where two or more products are used simultaneously (often including stimulants or products falsely claiming to protect the liver). This practice increases the risk of serious and life-threatening reactions.

WHAT TO DO

If you are taking bodybuilding products that claim to contain steroids or steroid-like substances, the FDA recommends stopping immediately due to the significant health risks. The agency also advises:

- Consult your health-care provider about any bodybuilding products or ingredients you have used or plan to use, especially if you are unsure about their safety.
- Seek medical advice if you experience symptoms such as:
  - nausea
  - weakness
  - fatigue
  - fever
  - abdominal pain
  - chest pain
  - shortness of breath
  - jaundice (yellowing of the skin or eyes)
  - dark or discolored urine

REGULATORY ACTION

In addition to issuing warning letters, the FDA can take further regulatory and enforcement actions against sellers of these illegal products. However, this process can be challenging, particularly when sellers operate solely online. Firm names or websites may be easily changed, or products may be relabeled to avoid detection and deceive consumers.[1]

---

[1] "Caution: Bodybuilding Products Can Be Risky," U.S. Food and Drug Administration (FDA), May 11, 2022. Available online. URL: www.fda.gov/consumers/consumer-updates/caution-bodybuilding-products-can-be-risky. Accessed September 10, 2024.

Chapter 33 | Guide to Sports Injury Management

Chapter Contents
Section 33.1—Understanding and Managing Sports
              Injuries 279
Section 33.2—Diagnosis, Treatment, and Management
              of Sports Injuries 281
Section 33.3—Understanding and Managing Concussions
              in Teens 285

Section 33.1 | Understanding and Managing Sports Injuries

The term "sports injury" refers to injuries that most commonly occur during sports or exercise, but they are not limited to athletes. Those who do exercises can get sports injuries, and factory workers can get tennis elbow, painters may experience shoulder injuries, and gardeners may develop tendinitis, even without participating in sports. Ultimately, however, sports injuries refer to those that occur in active individuals. While adverse events sometimes occur during sports or exercise, most physical activity is safe for nearly everyone, and the health benefits far outweigh the risks.

COMMON SPORTS INJURIES
Most sports injuries involve musculoskeletal injuries. The joints are particularly susceptible, as they bear significant demands. Joints must provide both stability and flexibility and are complex structures with several interconnected parts.

CAUSES OF SPORTS INJURIES
An acute sports injury is caused by a force of impact greater than the body part can withstand, while a chronic injury typically results from repeating the same motion over time. Those who do exercises can get sports injuries, and sometimes, overuse injuries degrade tissues and joints, setting the stage for an acute injury.

WHO GETS SPORTS INJURIES?
Anyone can experience a sports injury, but certain factors increase the risk.
   Risk factors for sports injuries include:
- not using the correct exercise techniques
- overtraining, whether by training too often, too frequently, or for too long
- changing the intensity of physical activity too quickly
- playing the same sport year-round

Fitness and Exercise Sourcebook, Seventh Edition

- running or jumping on hard surfaces
- wearing shoes that do not provide adequate support
- not wearing proper equipment
- having a previous injury
- having certain anatomical features specific to each joint or poor flexibility
- taking medications, such as fluoroquinolones, a class of antibiotics linked to tendinitis and tendon rupture

The type of injury one is most vulnerable to depends on the type of activity, age, and sex.

TYPES OF SPORTS INJURIES

Sports injuries are divided into two broad categories: acute and chronic injuries. Acute injuries happen suddenly, such as when a person falls, receives a blow, or twists a joint. Chronic injuries usually result from overuse of one area of the body and develop gradually over time. Examples of acute injuries include sprains and dislocations, while common chronic injuries include shin splints and stress fractures.

In some cases, wear and tear from overuse injuries can set the stage for acute injuries.

SYMPTOMS OF SPORTS INJURIES

The symptoms of a sports injury vary depending on the type of injury.

Symptoms of acute injuries include:
- sudden, severe pain
- extreme swelling or bruising
- inability to bear weight on a leg, knee, ankle, or foot
- inability to move a joint normally
- extreme weakness in an injured limb
- a bone or joint visibly out of place

Symptoms of chronic injuries due to overuse include:
- pain during activity or exercise
- swelling and a dull ache at rest

TREATMENT FOR A SPORTS INJURY

Treatment for a sports injury depends on the type of injury. Those who do exercises can get sports injuries, and minor injuries can usually be treated at home by resting, icing, compressing, and elevating (R-I-C-E) the injured part of the body. For more serious injuries, it is necessary to see a health-care provider, and physical therapy may be recommended for rehabilitation. In some cases, surgery may be required. A rehabilitation program that includes exercise and other types of therapy is typically recommended before resuming the sport or activity that caused the injury.[1]

Section 33.2 | Diagnosis, Treatment, and Management of Sports Injuries

The term "sports injury" refers to injuries that most commonly occur during sports or exercise, but they are not limited to athletes. Those who engage in exercise or physical activities can sustain sports injuries, and factory workers can develop tennis elbow, painters may experience shoulder injuries, and gardeners may develop tendinitis, even without participating in sports. Ultimately, sports injuries refer to those that occur in active individuals. While adverse events sometimes happen during sports or exercise, most physical activity is safe for nearly everyone, and the health benefits far outweigh the risks.

DIAGNOSIS OF SPORTS INJURIES

Those who do exercises can get sports injuries. To diagnose a sports injury, a doctor will likely take several steps, including the following actions.
- Ask about the injury and how it happened.
- Ask about any recreational or occupational activities and whether the intensity level of these activities has recently changed.

---

[1] "Sports Injuries," National Institute of Arthritis and Musculoskeletal and Skin Diseases (NIAMS), September 2021. Available online. URL: www.niams.nih.gov/health-topics/sports-injuries#tab-overview. Accessed September 10, 2024.

- Examine the injured area.
- Order imaging tests such as x-rays or magnetic resonance imaging (MRI) scans to evaluate the bones and soft tissues.

WHO TREATS SPORTS INJURIES?

Sports injuries are typically treated by:
- emergency physicians, who care for patients in emergency rooms for serious injuries
- primary health-care providers, including family doctors, internists, and pediatricians

Other specialists who may be involved in treatment include:
- orthopedic surgeons, who diagnose and treat injuries to bones, joints, ligaments, tendons, muscles, and nerves
- pain management specialists, who evaluate and treat pain
- physiatrists, who specialize in the nonsurgical management of musculoskeletal conditions and can develop rehabilitation plans
- physical therapists, who help patients:
  - develop rehabilitation programs
  - strengthen muscles and joints
  - prevent further injury
- sports medicine specialists, who work with athletes and others with musculoskeletal injuries

TREATMENT OF SPORTS INJURIES

It is important not to "work through" the pain of an injury, whether acute or from overuse. If pain occurs during a particular movement or activity, stop immediately. Continuing the activity may cause further harm.

The goals of treatment for a sports injury are to recover the injured part of the body and prevent future injuries.

Treatment for Serious Injuries
It is necessary to see a health-care provider if symptoms of a serious injury are present. These symptoms include:
- severe pain, swelling, or bruising
- pain and swelling that do not go away after a few days
- inability to tolerate any weight on the area
- an obvious deformity

Treatment for serious injuries may include:
- **Immobilization**. Immediate immobilization is a common treatment for musculoskeletal sports injuries, often performed by an athletic trainer or paramedic. Immobilization limits movement in the area and allows blood to flow more directly to the injury (or the site of surgical repair). This reduces pain, swelling, and muscle spasms and aids in the healing process. Most individuals need immobilization for only a limited time. Devices used for immobilization include:
  - slings to immobilize the upper body, including the arms and shoulders
  - splints, braces, and casts to support and protect injured bones and soft tissue
- **Surgery**. Surgery may be required to repair torn connective tissues or realign fractured bones. The vast majority of musculoskeletal sports injuries do not require surgery.

Treatment for Minor Injuries
If there are no symptoms of a serious injury, it is generally safe to treat the injury at home initially. However, if pain or other symptoms persist or worsen, it is important to consult a health-care provider. Use the R-I-C-E method to relieve pain, reduce inflammation, and speed healing:
- **Rest**. Limit activities involving the injured area for at least a day or two. Avoid putting weight on or using the injured joint or limb.

- **Ice**. Apply an ice pack to the injured area for 20 minutes at a time, four to eight times a day. Use a cold pack, ice bag, or plastic bag filled with crushed ice wrapped in a towel. Avoid applying ice for more than 20 minutes to prevent cold injury and frostbite.
- **Compression**. Keeping pressure on the injured area may help reduce swelling. Use an elastic bandage, but avoid wrapping it so tightly that it cuts off circulation.
- **Elevation**. If possible, elevate the injured ankle, knee, elbow, or wrist on a pillow above the level of the heart to help decrease swelling.

Other treatments may include over-the-counter (OTC) anti-inflammatory medications, which can help reduce pain and swelling.

REHABILITATION

After the injury heals, completing a rehabilitation program may be necessary before returning to the activity that caused the injury. A physical therapist or physiatrist will create a plan aimed at rebuilding strength and range of motion in the injured area, as well as easing any residual pain. Most rehabilitation plans include exercises performed both at home and in the therapist's office. The therapist may also use cold, heat, ultrasound, aquatic, or massage therapy to treat the injured area. A rehabilitation program helps individuals return to their previous level of activity and reduces the likelihood of re-injury.

LIVING WITH SPORTS INJURIES

Most sports injuries respond well to treatment and rehabilitation, enabling a return to normal activities. If pain persists, seeking help is essential. A primary health-care provider can manage most injury-related issues and may refer patients to an orthopedic surgeon, sports medicine specialist, or pain management specialist.

Once an injury heals, continuing regular exercise is important.

To avoid injury, you can take several precautions, including the following actions.
- Choose activities appropriate for your fitness level and gradually increase intensity.
- Use proper equipment and technique.
- Learn to identify injuries early and treat minor ones at home.
- Seek medical care when needed.

By following these steps, you can enjoy the health benefits of regular exercise while minimizing the risk of serious injury.[1]

Section 33.3 | Understanding and Managing Concussions in Teens

WHAT IS A CONCUSSION?

A concussion is a type of traumatic brain injury (TBI) caused by a bump, blow, or jolt to the head, or by a hit to the body that causes the head and brain to move quickly back and forth. Those who do exercises can get sports injuries such as concussions. This rapid movement can cause the brain to bounce around or twist inside the skull, leading to chemical changes in the brain and, in some cases, stretching and damaging brain cells.

HOW CAN TEENS STAY SAFE?

Sports are a great way for teens to stay healthy and can help them excel in school. To help reduce the risk of concussions or other serious brain injuries, consider the following:
- Create a culture of safety for the team:
  - Work with the coach to teach ways to lower the chances of concussion.

---

[1] "Sports Injuries: Diagnosis, Treatment, and Steps to Take," National Institute of Arthritis and Musculoskeletal and Skin Diseases (NIAMS), September 2021. Available online. URL: www.niams.nih.gov/health-topics/sports-injuries/diagnosis-treatment-and-steps-to-take. Accessed September 10, 2024.

- Emphasize the importance of reporting concussions and allowing time for recovery.
- Ensure teens follow the coach's safety rules and the rules of the sport.
- Encourage teens to practice good sportsmanship at all times.
- Use helmets when appropriate:
  - Teach teens to wear helmets for sports or activities that require them to help reduce the chances of serious brain or head injuries. There is no "concussion-proof" helmet, so it is still important to avoid hits to the head, even when wearing a helmet.

HOW CAN YOU SPOT A POSSIBLE CONCUSSION?

Teens who do exercises can also get sports injuries, and those who show or report one or more of the following signs and symptoms after a bump, blow, or jolt to the head or body—or who simply say they "do not feel right"—may have a concussion or another serious brain injury.

Signs observed by parents:
- appears dazed or stunned
- forgets instructions, seems confused about an assignment or position, or is unsure of the game, score, or opponent
- moves clumsily
- answers questions slowly
- loses consciousness (even briefly)
- shows changes in mood, behavior, or personality
- cannot recall events before or after a hit or fall

Symptoms reported by teens:
- headache or "pressure" in the head
- nausea or vomiting
- balance problems or dizziness
- double or blurry vision
- sensitivity to light or noise
- feeling sluggish, hazy, foggy, or groggy

- confusion, difficulty concentrating, or memory problems
- just not "feeling right" or feeling down

CONCUSSIONS AFFECT EACH TEEN DIFFERENTLY

While most teens with a concussion feel better within a couple of weeks, some may have symptoms that last for months or longer. It is important to consult a health-care provider if symptoms persist or worsen after a return to normal activities.

SERIOUS DANGER SIGNS TO LOOK OUT FOR

In rare cases, a dangerous collection of blood (hematoma) may form on the brain after a bump, blow, or jolt to the head or body, which can put pressure on the brain. Call 911 or take your teen to the emergency department immediately if they exhibit any of these danger signs:
- one pupil larger than the other
- drowsiness or inability to wake up
- a headache that worsens and does not go away
- slurred speech, weakness, numbness, or decreased coordination
- repeated vomiting or nausea, convulsions, or seizures
- unusual behavior, confusion, restlessness, or agitation
- loss of consciousness (even brief unconsciousness should be taken seriously)

Teens who do exercises can get sports injuries, and those who continue to play with concussion symptoms or return to play too soon—before the brain has healed—are at a higher risk of another concussion. A repeat concussion during recovery from the first injury can have serious consequences, potentially affecting the teen for life or even being fatal.[1]

---

[1] "A Fact Sheet for High School Parents," Centers for Disease Control and Prevention (CDC), January 2019. Available online. URL: www.cdc.gov/heads-up/media/pdfs/highschoolsports/parents_fact_sheet-a.pdf. Accessed September 10, 2024.

Chapter 34 | **Exercising Outdoors in Polluted Air**

Science has shown the benefits of exercise and physical activity. But what about exercising outside when air pollution levels are high, such as during a wildfire or on a hot, sunny day with elevated ozone levels?

The answer is that it depends. The level of air pollution, a person's health status, and the duration and intensity of exercise are all important factors to consider. Physical activity has long been recognized as essential to health and is recommended by the U.S. Department of Health and Human Services (HHS). The 2018 HHS guidelines refer to the U.S. Environmental Protection Agency's (EPA) Air Quality Index (AQI) for guidance about exercising or engaging in physical activity when air pollution is in the forecast.

EPA researchers are working to improve knowledge about the relationship between exercise and air pollution, which has not been an active area of research until recently. In 2010, the Centers for Disease Control and Prevention (CDC) held a workshop to review the state of the science and existing public health guidance on physical activity and outdoor air pollution exposure. The international experts attending the workshop recommended further research to inform future public health guidance.

Since then, the study of the potential health effects of air pollution during exercise has gained popularity, especially in the last five years, says Stephanie DeFlorio-Barker, an epidemiologist in EPA's Office of Research and Development. DeFlorio-Barker and her colleagues conducted a systematic scientific review of the literature published between 2000 and 2020 on the short-term health effects of air pollution exposure during outdoor exercise.

They found 25 studies and selected 16 that met their criteria for examining short-term effects and including four distinct study groups:
1. exercising in clean air
2. exercising in polluted air
3. resting in clean air
4. resting in polluted air

According to DeFlorio-Barker, these criteria allowed for a more consistent and scientifically rigorous comparison of results. However, the review presented challenges due to wide variations in research methods, the diversity of study groups, and the types of health effects studied.

"The main question we were trying to answer in the review is: Are there worsening health effects among individuals while exercising in polluted air?" says DeFlorio-Barker.

Nine of the sixteen studies reviewed demonstrated that exercising outdoors in polluted air results in short-term (temporary) health effects, with lung function impairments being the most observed. The other seven studies, which examined different health effects, such as inflammation and blood pressure, found no significant effects.

The study, published in the journal *Preventive Medicine*, showed that healthy individuals who engaged in moderate- to high-intensity exercise outdoors in low or high levels of air pollution experienced fewer health effects compared to those doing low-intensity exercise. For people with preexisting conditions such as respiratory or cardiovascular disease, even low-intensity activities such as walking may intensify the negative effects of air pollution, the study suggests.

"Personally, I expected to see that high-intensity exercise resulted in worsening effects due to the increased dose of air pollution, but really we found the opposite," DeFlorio-Barker says. The findings indicate a need for further study, she adds.[1]

---

[1] "Should You Exercise outside in Air Pollution?" U.S. Environmental Protection Agency (EPA), September 4, 2024. Available online. URL: www.epa.gov/sciencematters/should-you-exercise-outside-air-pollution. Accessed September 10, 2024.

Part 6 | Physical Fitness for Health Conditions

Chapter 35 | Physical Activity for Chronic Conditions

Regular physical activity can promote improved quality of life (QOL) for people with chronic conditions and reduce the risk of developing new conditions. The type and amount of physical activity should be determined by a person's abilities and the severity of the chronic condition.

PHYSICAL ACTIVITY IN ADULTS WITH OSTEOARTHRITIS

Osteoarthritis is a common condition in older adults, and people can live many years with it. People with osteoarthritis are often concerned that physical activity can worsen their condition. Osteoarthritis can be painful and cause fatigue, making it difficult to begin or maintain regular physical activity. Yet, people with this condition should engage in regular physical activity to lower their risk of developing other chronic diseases, such as heart disease or type 2 diabetes, and to help maintain a healthy body weight.

Physical activity provides both preventive and therapeutic health benefits for people with osteoarthritis. Strong scientific evidence indicates that both aerobic activity and muscle-strengthening exercises offer therapeutic benefits. Regular physical activity improves pain, physical function, QOL, and mental health for adults with osteoarthritis. When done safely, physical activity does not worsen the disease or pain. Evidence also shows that the benefits of physical activity can continue even after stopping a physical activity program.

People with osteoarthritis should match the type and amount of physical activity to their abilities and the severity of their condition. Most people can tolerate moderate-intensity activity for 150 minutes a week or more, such as being active three to five days a week for 30–60 minutes per session. Walking up to 10,000 steps per day does not appear to worsen knee osteoarthritis. Some people with osteoarthritis can safely exceed 150 minutes of moderate-intensity activity each week and may be able to tolerate vigorous-intensity activity. Health-care professionals typically advise people with osteoarthritis to engage in low effect, non-painful activities that have a low risk of joint injury. Swimming, walking, tai chi, and muscle-strengthening exercises are good examples of such activities.

PHYSICAL ACTIVITY IN ADULTS WITH TYPE 2 DIABETES

Physical activity in adults with type 2 diabetes highlights the importance of being active for those with chronic diseases. Physical activity has therapeutic effects, reduces comorbidities, and helps prevent risk factors that contribute to the progression of type 2 diabetes. Therefore, in addition to diabetes-specific benefits, physical activity is routinely recommended to reduce the risk of other diseases and promote a healthy body weight.

Strong scientific evidence shows that physical activity protects against heart disease, the leading cause of death in people with type 2 diabetes, and can reduce the risk of death by 30–40 percent. Physical activity helps reduce the risk factors associated with heart disease and the progression of type 2 diabetes by lowering high blood pressure (HBP), body weight, blood lipids (cholesterol), and hemoglobin A1c levels in people with type 2 diabetes. The beneficial effects on blood glucose (as indicated by hemoglobin A1c) may also reduce other complications of type 2 diabetes. Moderate-intensity activity for at least 150 minutes a week, plus two days of muscle-strengthening activities, can substantially lower the risk of heart disease. Those who move toward 300 minutes or more of moderate-intensity activity per week experience even greater benefits.

Adults with chronic conditions should work with a health-care professional or physical activity specialist to adapt physical activity to their condition. For example, people with diabetes must be especially careful about monitoring their blood glucose, choosing appropriate footwear, and avoiding injury to their feet.

PHYSICAL ACTIVITY IN ADULTS WITH HYPERTENSION

Hypertension is one of the most common, costly, and preventable cardiovascular disease risk factors. It is the most prevalent chronic condition among adults. Physical activity provides therapeutic benefits for people with hypertension by helping reduce blood pressure and lowering the risk of cardiovascular disease mortality.

Both aerobic and muscle-strengthening activities benefit people with hypertension. Physical activity has greater benefits for people with hypertension than for those with normal blood pressure. Moderate-intensity activity for about 90 minutes a week, or the equivalent amount of vigorous-intensity activity, can substantially lower the risk of heart disease. Increasing physical activity beyond these amounts leads to even greater benefits. People with hypertension should work with their health-care provider as they increase their physical activity, as medication adjustments may be needed.

PHYSICAL ACTIVITY IN ADULT CANCER SURVIVORS

Earlier detection of cancer and modern improved treatments mean that more than 15.5 million cancer survivors are living in the United States today. This growing population faces unique challenges, including the risk of recurrent cancer, death from cancer or other causes, the development of other chronic diseases, and the worsening of physical functioning and QOL.

Cancer survivors should engage in regular physical activity for its many health benefits. For adults with breast, colorectal, or prostate cancer, greater amounts of physical activity after diagnosis substantially lower the risk of dying from cancer. For adults with breast and colorectal cancer, increased physical activity also lowers the risk of dying from any cause. Physically active cancer survivors experience a better QOL, improved fitness and physical function, and less fatigue. Physical activity also helps reduce the adverse effects of cancer treatment. Some cancer survivors are at increased risk of heart disease, and physical activity can help reduce this risk.[1]

---

[1] Office of Disease Prevention and Health Promotion (ODPHP), "Current Guidelines," U.S. Department of Health and Human Services (HHS), August 24, 2021. Available online. URL: https://health.gov/our-work/nutrition-physical-activity/physical-activity-guidelines/current-guidelines. Accessed September 10, 2024.

Chapter 36 | Fitness for People with Disabilities

Chapter Contents
Section 36.1—Healthy Living for People with Disabilities.......299
Section 36.2—Staying Active with a Disability...........................301

Section 36.1 | **Healthy Living for People with Disabilities**

DISABILITY AND HEALTH: HEALTHY LIVING

People with disabilities need health care and health programs for the same reasons as everyone else—to stay well, active, and engaged in their communities.

Having a disability does not mean a person is not healthy or cannot be healthy. Being healthy means the same thing for everyone—getting and staying well so we can lead full, active lives. This involves having the tools and information to make healthy choices and knowing how to prevent illness.

For people with disabilities, being healthy also means recognizing that health problems related to a disability can be treated. These problems, called "secondary conditions," can include pain, depression, and an increased risk for certain illnesses.

To stay healthy, people with disabilities need health care that addresses their needs as a whole person, not just as a person with a disability. Most people, with or without disabilities, can maintain their health by learning about and adopting healthy lifestyles.

LEADING A LONG AND HEALTHY LIFE

Although people with disabilities may face greater challenges in getting and staying healthy than people without disabilities, there are steps everyone can take to achieve and maintain good health.

- Be physically active every day.
- Eat healthy foods in healthy portions.
- Limit sun exposure.
- Do not smoke.
- Use medications wisely.
- If you drink alcoholic beverages, do so in moderation.
- Seek help for substance abuse.
- Stay connected with family and friends.
- If you need assistance, consult your health-care professional.

GETTING THE BEST POSSIBLE HEALTH CARE

People with disabilities must receive the care and services necessary to maintain their health.

If you have a disability, there are steps you can take to ensure you are getting the best possible health care:

- Know your body, how you feel when you are well, and when you are not.
- Communicate openly with your health-care professional about your concerns.
- Find health-care professionals you are comfortable with in your area.
- Ensure you can physically access your health-care professional's office, including ramps or elevators if you use an assistive device such as a wheelchair or scooter.
- Check whether your health-care professional's office has the equipment you need, such as an accessible scale or examining table.
- Ask for help from the office staff if necessary.
- Think about your questions and concerns before your visit so that you are prepared.
- Bring your health records with you.
- Bring a friend if you are concerned you might forget your questions or the health-care professional's advice.
- Write down, or have someone write down for you, what your health-care professional says.

PHYSICAL ACTIVITY

Adults of all shapes, sizes, and abilities can benefit from being physically active, including those with disabilities. To achieve significant health benefits, all adults should engage in both aerobic and muscle-strengthening physical activities. Regular aerobic physical activity increases heart and lung function, improves daily living activities and independence, decreases the risk of developing chronic diseases, and enhances mental health.

Adults with disabilities should aim for at least 150 minutes per week of moderate-intensity aerobic physical activity (e.g., brisk walking, wheeling oneself in a wheelchair) or at least 75 minutes per week of vigorous-intensity aerobic physical activity (e.g., jogging, wheelchair basketball), or a combination of both moderate- and vigorous-intensity aerobic activities each week. A rule of thumb is that one minute of vigorous-intensity activity equals about two minutes of moderate-intensity activity. They should avoid inactivity, as some physical activity is better than none.

Muscle-strengthening activities should involve moderate and high intensity, engaging all major muscle groups on two or more days per week (e.g., using resistance bands, adapted yoga) to gain additional health benefits. All children and adolescents should participate in 60 minutes or more of physical activity each day.

If a person with a disability is unable to meet the physical activity guidelines, they should engage in regular physical activity based on their abilities and avoid inactivity. Adults with disabilities should consult their health-care provider about the appropriate types and amounts of physical activity for their abilities.

TIPS FOR GETTING FIT
- Talk to your doctor about how much and what types of physical activity are right for you.
- Find opportunities to increase physical activity regularly in ways that meet your needs and abilities.
- Start slowly, based on your abilities and fitness level (e.g., be active for at least 10 minutes at a time, gradually increasing activity over several weeks, if necessary).
- Avoid inactivity. Some activity is better than none![1]

Section 36.2 | **Staying Active with a Disability**

HEALTH BENEFITS OF PHYSICAL ACTIVITY FOR PEOPLE WITH DISABILITIES

Everyone needs physical activity for good health. However, less than half of U.S. adults with serious difficulty walking or climbing stairs (mobility disability) report engaging in aerobic physical

---

[1] National Center on Birth Defects and Developmental Disabilities (NCBDDD), "Disability and Health Healthy Living," Centers for Disease Control and Prevention (CDC), May 2, 2024. Available online. URL: www.cdc.gov/ncbddd/disabilityandhealth/healthyliving.html. Accessed September 10, 2024.

activity. For those who are active, walking is the most common physical activity. Decide how much physical activity is right for you and your fitness level. Choose an activity you enjoy—such as gardening, doing household chores, wheeling yourself in your wheelchair, walking briskly, or dancing—and find ways to incorporate it into your daily routine. Getting active can help you:
- strengthen your heart
- build strong muscles
- lower stress
- boost your mood
- improve symptoms of anxiety or depression

TIPS FOR INCORPORATING PHYSICAL ACTIVITY FOR PEOPLE WITH DISABILITIES

- Choose activities that make your heart beat faster, such as walking briskly, chair boxing, swimming, or raking leaves.
- If possible, aim for 150 minutes per week of moderate-intensity aerobic activity.
- Start slowly and do what you can—even five minutes of physical activity offers real health benefits, and you can gradually build up to more over time.

MUSCLE-STRENGTHENING ACTIVITIES FOR PEOPLE WITH DISABILITIES

- Muscle-strengthening activities include activities such as push-ups or lifting weights. Choose activities that work for you.
- You may need assistance with certain muscle-strengthening activities. Consult your doctor or a trained physical activity specialist if you feel you need help.
- If possible, work on the muscles you use less often.

STAYING MOTIVATED AND BUILDING A ROUTINE

- Try different activities until you find something you enjoy—that way, you are more likely to stick with it!

Fitness for People with Disabilities

- Some people find that getting active with friends helps them stay motivated, while others prefer to exercise alone. It is all about what works best for you.
- If having a routine is helpful, plan activities ahead of time. For instance, you could take a weekly fitness class or visit the park at the same time every day.
- Consider reaching out to a trained physical activity specialist, such as a physical therapist or certified exercise professional. They can help you plan a routine that fits your needs and helps you feel your best—physically and mentally.
- If you do not meet your physical activity goal, do not give up—you can try again tomorrow.

CONSULTING YOUR DOCTOR

Consider discussing with your doctor the types and amounts of physical activity that are right for you. You can ask questions such as:
- What activities would you recommend for me?
- Can you refer me to a trained physical activity specialist, such as a physical therapist or personal trainer?
- Can you recommend a gym or recreation center near me with experience working with people with similar disabilities?
- If you are taking any medicine, ask if it could affect how your body responds to physical activity.[1]

---

[1] Office of Disease Prevention and Health Promotion (ODPHP), "Stay Active with a Disability: Quick Tips," U.S. Department of Health and Human Services (HHS), February 14, 2024. Available online. URL: https://health.gov/myhealthfinder/health-conditions/obesity/stay-active-disability-quick-tips. Accessed September 10, 2024.

Chapter 37 | Fitness for Overweight Individuals

Chapter Contents
Section 37.1—Overweight, Obesity, and the Role of
 Physical Activity 307
Section 37.2—Physical Activity for People of All Sizes 309

Section 37.1 | Overweight, Obesity, and the Role of Physical Activity

OVERWEIGHT AND OBESITY
People whose weight is higher than what is considered healthy for their height are described as overweight or obese. Overweight and obesity can increase the risk for many health problems.

BODY MASS INDEX
Overweight and obesity are defined by body mass index (BMI). BMI is a measurement that uses weight and height to estimate overweight and obesity. Table 37.1 shows BMI ranges for overweight and obesity in adults aged 20 and older.

Table 37.1. BMI of Adults Aged 20 and Older

BMI	Category
18.5–24.9	Healthy weight
25.0–29.9	Overweight
30.0–39.9	Obesity
40.0 and above	Severe obesity

PREVALENCE OF OVERWEIGHT AND OBESITY
Overweight and obesity are common among U.S. adults aged 20 and older. According to estimates based on data from the 2017 to 2018 National Health and Nutrition Examination Survey (NHANES):
- Nearly one in three adults (30.7%) are overweight.
- More than 2 in 5 adults (42.4%) have obesity, including about 1 in 11 adults (9.2%) with severe obesity.
- Nearly three in four adults (73.1%) are either overweight or obese.

DIFFERENCES BY SEX
Men are more likely than women to be overweight or obese. Among adults aged 20 and older, 77.1 percent of men and 69.4 percent of women are overweight or obese. However, severe obesity, or having a BMI greater than 40, is more common among women (11.5%) than men (6.9%).

DIFFERENCES BY RACE AND ETHNICITY
Overweight and obesity rates also vary among racial and ethnic groups. According to 2017–2018 NHANES data, obesity affects:
- nearly one in two non-Hispanic Black adults (49.6%)
- more than two in five Hispanic adults (44.8%)
- more than two in five non-Hispanic white adults (42.2%)
- more than one in six non-Hispanic Asian adults (17.4%)

VARIATIONS AMONG OTHER GROUPS
Overweight and obesity also vary among other groups. For example, obesity is more common among people in rural areas than among those who live in urban areas.

HEALTH BENEFITS OF PHYSICAL ACTIVITY
Physical activity can help you lose excess weight and maintain a healthy weight. Being active is also linked to numerous other health benefits. Regular aerobic activity can prevent and reduce health problems, such as high blood pressure (HBP) and high blood glucose (blood sugar), and improve mental health.

The *Physical Activity Guidelines for Americans, 2nd edition* recommends that healthy adults:
- Engage in moderate-intensity aerobic activity, such as brisk walking or dancing, for at least 150 minutes a week. Moderate-intensity activity makes your heart beat faster and your breathing harder, but it should not be overly strenuous.
- Participate in muscle-strengthening activities that involve all major muscle groups on two or more days a week.

Fitness for Overweight Individuals

Adults with chronic health conditions or disabilities who cannot meet these guidelines should still engage in regular physical activities they can do safely. If you have a health condition such as heart disease, HBP, or diabetes, consult your health-care professional before starting regular physical activity. They can help you find safe activities that will benefit you the most.

Regular physical activity can also help you maintain weight loss. To prevent weight regain, aim for at least 300 minutes a week of moderate-intensity physical activity. Make physical activity a lifelong habit.[1]

Section 37.2 | Physical Activity for People of All Sizes

Physical activity may seem challenging if you are overweight. You may become short of breath or tired quickly. Finding or affording the right clothes and equipment may be frustrating, or you may not feel comfortable working out in front of others. The good news is that you can overcome these challenges. Not only can you be active at any size, but you can also have fun and feel good at the same time.

CAN ANYONE BE ACTIVE?

Research strongly shows that physical activity is safe for almost everyone. The health benefits of physical activity far outweigh the risks.

The activities discussed here are safe for most people. If you have difficulty moving or staying steady on your feet, or if you become easily short of breath, talk with a health-care professional before you start. You should also consult with a health-care professional if you

---

[1] "Understanding Adult Overweight and Obesity," National Institute of Diabetes and Digestive and Kidney Diseases (NIDDK), May 2023. Available online. URL: www.niddk.nih.gov/health-information/weight-management/adult-overweight-obesity/definition-facts. Accessed September 10, 2024.

are unsure about your health, have concerns that physical activity may be unsafe for you, or have:
- a chronic disease such as diabetes, high blood pressure (HBP), or heart disease
- a bone or joint problem—such as in your back, knee, or hip—that could worsen with increased physical activity

WHY SHOULD YOU BE ACTIVE?

Being active may help you live longer and protect you from serious health problems such as type 2 diabetes, heart disease, stroke, and certain types of cancer. Regular physical activity is linked to many health benefits, including:
- lower blood pressure and blood glucose levels
- healthy bones, muscles, and joints
- a strong heart and lungs
- better sleep at night and improved mood

WHAT DO YOU NEED TO KNOW ABOUT BECOMING ACTIVE?

Choosing physical activities that match your fitness level and health goals can help you stay motivated and avoid injury. You may feel minor discomfort or muscle soreness when you first start, but this should subside as your body adapts to the activity. However, if you experience nausea or pain, you may be overdoing it. Scale back your activity and gradually increase your level of effort.

If you have been inactive, start slowly and see how you feel. Gradually increase the duration and frequency of your activity. For guidance, consult a health-care professional or a certified fitness expert.

Here are some tips for staying safe during physical activity:
- Wear the proper safety gear, such as a bike helmet if you are bicycling.
- Make sure any sports equipment you use is in good condition and fits properly.
- Choose safe locations to be active, such as well-lit areas where others are around. Consider being active with a friend or group.

Fitness for Overweight Individuals

- Stay hydrated to replace fluids lost through sweat and to prevent overheating.
- If you are outdoors, protect yourself from the sun with sunscreen, a hat, or protective clothing.
- Dress in layers to stay warm in cold or windy weather.

If you do not feel well, stop your activity. Seek help immediately if you experience:
- pain, tightness, or pressure in your chest, neck, shoulder, or arm
- extreme shortness of breath
- dizziness or nausea

WHAT KINDS OF ACTIVITIES CAN YOU DO?
You do not need to be an athlete or have special skills to incorporate physical activity into your life. Many daily activities, such as walking your dog or climbing stairs, can improve your health.

Try different activities you enjoy. If you find an activity fun, you are more likely to stick with it. Anything that gets you moving, even for a few minutes at a time, is a good step toward better fitness.
- walking
- dancing
- bicycling
- water workouts
- strength training
- mind and body exercises
- daily activities

WHERE CAN YOU BE ACTIVE?
You can find many enjoyable places to be active. Having several options may help prevent boredom. Consider these choices:
- Join or take a class at a local fitness, recreation, or community center.
- Enjoy the outdoors by hiking or walking in a safe local park, neighborhood, or mall.
- Work out at home with a fitness video or by using a fitness channel on your TV, tablet, or other mobile device.

Fitness and Exercise Sourcebook, Seventh Edition

HOW CAN YOU STICK WITH YOUR PHYSICAL ACTIVITY PLAN?

Staying committed to a physical activity plan can be challenging, but online tools such as the National Institutes of Health (NIH) Body Weight Planner (www.niddk.nih.gov/health-information/weight-management/body-weight-planner) can help. This tool allows you to customize your calorie and physical activity plans to meet your personal goals over time.

You can also use fitness apps to track your progress on a computer, smartphone, or other mobile device.

Wearable devices such as pedometers and fitness trackers can help you count steps, calories, and activity minutes. These devices may also assist you in setting goals and monitoring progress. Most trackers can be worn on your wrist like a watch or clipped to your clothing.

Keeping an activity journal is another way to stay motivated and on track with your fitness goals.

- **Set goals**. Instead of vague goals such as "I will be more active," set specific goals such as "I will take a walk after lunch at least two days a week." Start with small, achievable goals to build a new habit. A short-term goal may be walking 5–10 minutes five days a week. A long-term goal could be achieving at least 150 minutes of moderate-intensity physical activity a week.
- **Get support**. Ask a family member or friend to be active with you. A workout buddy can make activities more enjoyable and provide encouragement to meet your goals.
- **Track progress**. Even if you do not notice immediate changes, you may be pleasantly surprised when you look back at where you started. Making regular activity a part of your life is a big step. Praise yourself for every goal you meet.
- **Review your goals**. Did you achieve your goals? If not, why? Are your goals realistic? Identify any obstacles and brainstorm ways to overcome them. Ask a friend or family member for support.
- **Pick nonfood rewards**. Whether your goal is to be active for 15 minutes a day, walk farther than last

Fitness for Overweight Individuals

week, or stay positive, recognizing your efforts is key to staying motivated. Treat yourself to rewards such as new music or workout gear to celebrate your progress.
- **Be patient**. Do not get discouraged by setbacks. If you cannot reach your goal immediately, or only manage to stick to your goals part of the week, remember that building new habits takes time.
- **Look ahead**. Focus on future improvements rather than past difficulties. Celebrate your progress and keep moving forward.

Most importantly, do not give up. Every movement, no matter how small, is a positive step toward better health.[1]

---

[1] "Staying Active at Any Size," National Institute of Diabetes and Digestive and Kidney Diseases (NIDDK), July 2016. Available online. URL: www.niddk.nih.gov/health-information/weight-management/staying-active-at-any-size. Accessed September 10, 2024.

Chapter 38 | Cardiac Rehabilitation for Heart Health Recovery

Each year, about 800,000 people in the United States experience a heart attack, and approximately one in four of them have had a heart attack before. If you have a heart attack or other heart problem, cardiac rehabilitation is an important part of your recovery. It can help you recover from a heart issue and also reduce the risk of future heart problems.

WHAT IS CARDIAC REHABILITATION?
Cardiac rehabilitation is a supervised program that includes:
- physical activity
- education on healthy living, such as eating a balanced diet, taking prescribed medication, and quitting smoking
- counseling to manage stress and improve mental health

A team of professionals, including your health-care providers, exercise and nutrition specialists, physical therapists, and counselors, may guide you through cardiac rehabilitation.

WHO NEEDS CARDIAC REHABILITATION?
Anyone who has had a heart problem, such as a heart attack, heart failure, or heart surgery, can benefit from cardiac rehabilitation. Studies show that cardiac rehabilitation helps men and women of all ages with mild, moderate, or severe heart conditions.

However, some individuals are less likely to start or complete a cardiac rehabilitation program.
- **Women**. Studies indicate that women, especially minority women, are less likely than men to begin or complete cardiac rehabilitation. This may be because doctors are less likely to recommend the program to women.
- **Older adults**. Older adults are also less likely to participate in cardiac rehabilitation after a heart event. They may feel unable to engage in physical activity due to age or other conditions, such as arthritis, that make exercise more difficult. Cardiac rehabilitation can be especially beneficial for older adults by improving strength and mobility, making daily tasks easier.

HOW CARDIAC REHABILITATION HELPS
Cardiac rehabilitation provides numerous short- and long-term health benefits, including:
- strengthening the heart and body after a heart attack
- relieving symptoms of heart problems, such as chest pain
- promoting healthier habits, such as increasing physical activity, quitting smoking, and following a heart-healthy diet
- reducing stress
- improving mood, especially since people are more prone to depression after a heart attack; cardiac rehabilitation can help prevent or alleviate depression
- increasing energy and strength to make daily activities, such as carrying groceries or climbing stairs, easier
- encouraging adherence to prescribed medications, lowering the risk of future heart problems
- reducing the likelihood of future illness and death from heart disease

WHERE TO GET CARDIAC REHABILITATION

Cardiac rehabilitation programs may take place in a hospital, rehabilitation center, or even at home. The program can begin while you are still in the hospital or soon after you are discharged.

Most cardiac rehabilitation programs last about three months, but they can range from two to eight months.

Talk to your doctor about cardiac rehabilitation. Many insurance plans, including Medicaid and Medicare, cover the program if you have a doctor's referral.[1]

---

[1] "How Cardiac Rehabilitation Can Help Heal Your Heart," Centers for Disease Control and Prevention (CDC), May 24, 2024. Available online. URL: www.cdc.gov/heart-disease/about/cardiac-rehabilitation-treatment.html. Accessed September 10, 2024.

Chapter 39 | Fitness for Bone Disorders

Chapter Contents
Section 39.1—Managing Arthritis with Physical Activity........321
Section 39.2—Preventing Osteoporosis through Exercise.......324
Section 39.3—Managing Osteogenesis Imperfecta....................327

Section 39.1 | Managing Arthritis with Physical Activity

WHAT IS ARTHRITIS?
Arthritis is a general term for conditions that affect the joints, tissues around joints, and other connective tissues. There are more than 100 types of arthritis.

RISK FACTORS
Certain behaviors and characteristics can increase your chances of developing arthritis. Many of these risk factors are within your control, including:
- smoking
- having overweight or obesity
- joint injuries, such as those from sports, falls, and accidents
- work-related activities that lead to joint injury, such as bending, squatting, and other repetitive motions

SYMPTOMS AND DIAGNOSIS
Symptoms vary depending on the type of arthritis but often include joint pain and stiffness.

Health-care providers can diagnose arthritis by:
- reviewing your health and family history
- performing a physical exam
- taking x-rays
- conducting lab tests (as needed)

Once you know the type of arthritis you have, you can work with your provider to determine the best ways to manage and treat it.

MANAGING YOUR ARTHRITIS
It is important to manage arthritis symptoms to:
- prevent or delay the progression of the condition and avoid disability
- reduce pain
- improve your overall health and well-being

WAYS TO MANAGE ARTHRITIS
Here are five ways to manage arthritis and its symptoms:
- Learn self-management skills.
- Be physically active.
- Manage your weight.
- Protect your joints.
- Talk to your health-care provider if you have symptoms.

TREATMENT OPTIONS
There is no cure for arthritis, but it can be treated and managed. Treatment options vary depending on the type of arthritis and may include:
- over-the-counter (OTC) medicines
- physical therapy
- prescription medicines
- surgery, if needed

Your provider will discuss these and other treatment options that are appropriate for your arthritis type and personal needs.

PHYSICAL ACTIVITY AND ARTHRITIS
Physical activity can help people with arthritis reduce joint pain, improve function, and boost mood. Managing your symptoms through physical activity can result in better health and quality of life (QOL).

Be Active to Manage Arthritis
Everyone should aim to move more and sit less throughout the day to maintain good health.

Recommended Mix of Physical Activity
Adults, including those with arthritis, need a mix of activities to stay healthy. It is recommended that adults do:
- at least 150 minutes a week of moderate-intensity aerobic activity, such as brisk walking

Fitness for Bone Disorders

- at least two days a week of muscle-strengthening activities, such as those that make your muscles work harder than usual

Older adults should aim for a mix of aerobic, muscle-strengthening, and balance activities each week. You can break up your physical activity into short sessions. Just 5–10 minutes at a time is beneficial. As long as you get the recommended amount each week, you will gain the full benefits of physical activity.

Joint-Friendly Physical Activities
The best activities to choose are those that:
- are fun
- are easy to access
- cause little or no pain
- are sustainable over time

Joint-friendly physical activities that put no or low stress on the joints include:
- brisk walking
- cycling
- light gardening
- dancing
- tai chi
- swimming
- water exercises, such as shoulder shrugs and ankle circles in the water

For strength training, choose weights or resistance bands that do not cause joint pain. As your body adjusts to an activity, you can increase the difficulty in small increments over time.

Starting Physical Activity
When starting or increasing physical activity, begin slowly and pay attention to how your body feels. It is normal to experience some pain, stiffness, or swelling after starting a new physical activity program.

Over time, arthritis-related joint pain from physical activity should improve. If it does not, contact your health-care provider.

When to Talk to Your Provider
BEFORE STARTING PHYSICAL ACTIVITY
If possible, talk to a health-care provider before beginning physical activity for personalized recommendations. People with arthritis may benefit from seeing a physical therapist when starting a new physical activity routine.

AFTER STARTING YOUR PHYSICAL ACTIVITY ROUTINE
Contact your health-care provider if pain or other symptoms are severe after starting a physical activity program.[1]

Section 39.2 | Preventing Osteoporosis through Exercise

EXERCISE AND BONE HEALTH
As people age, their risk of osteoporosis rises. Osteoporosis is a disease that causes bones to become weak and brittle, increasing the risk of fractures (broken bones). Older adults also tend to lose muscle (a condition called "sarcopenia"). Strong muscles are essential for balance and reduce the risk of falls and broken bones.

Exercise at any age, for both adults and children, offers many benefits for bone health, such as:
- building strong bones in children
- strengthening muscles and bones in both children and adults
- preventing bone loss in adults
- increasing bone density and replacing old bone with new bone
- improving balance and coordination

---

[1] "About Physical Activity and Arthritis," Centers for Disease Control and Prevention (CDC), February 14, 2024. Available online. URL: www.cdc.gov/arthritis/prevention/index.html. Accessed September 10, 2024.

Fitness for Bone Disorders

- helping prevent falls and fractures
- helping prevent osteoporosis

WHICH EXERCISES ARE BEST FOR KEEPING BONES HEALTHY?

If you have low bone density (sometimes called "osteopenia"), osteoporosis, or other physical limitations, talk to a health-care provider before starting an exercise program. They can help you choose types of physical activity that are safe for you and beneficial for your bone health.

A combination of the following types of exercise is best for building and maintaining healthy bones and preventing falls and fractures:

- **Weight-bearing exercises**. These exercises create a force on bones that makes them work harder. Examples include:
    - brisk walking (three to four miles per hour)
    - jogging or running
    - tennis, badminton, ping pong, pickleball, and other racket sports
    - climbing stairs
    - dancing
- **Resistance training exercises**. These exercises add resistance to movement, making muscles work harder and become stronger. They also put stress on bones, which helps strengthen them. Strength-training exercises can involve:
    - weight machines
    - free weights
    - resistance bands
    - use of your own body weight (such as pushups or pullups)
- **Balance training**. This is especially important for older adults. It improves balance and helps prevent falls. Examples include:
    - walking on an unstable surface (e.g., a foam mat or wobble board)
    - tai chi
    - walking backwards

Fitness and Exercise Sourcebook, Seventh Edition

- step-ups
- lunges
- shifting your body weight backward and forward while standing with both feet together or on one foot

HOW MUCH EXERCISE DO WE NEED TO KEEP BONES HEALTHY?

According to the U.S. Department of Health and Human Services (HHS), adults of all ages should aim for the following amounts of exercise to maintain bone health:

- **For all adults**. At least 150 minutes of moderate-intensity exercise per week, or at least 75 minutes of vigorous-intensity exercise per week. Additionally, muscle-strengthening activities of at least moderate intensity should be done at least twice a week for added benefit.
- **For older adults**. The weekly 150 minutes of exercise should include a mix of balance training, aerobic, and muscle-strengthening exercises. If they cannot do 150 minutes of moderate-intensity physical activity because of health limitations, they should be as physically active as their health allows.
- **For pregnant women and postpartum women**. Women should aim for at least 150 minutes per week of moderate-intensity exercise, ideally spread throughout the week. Pregnant women should consult a health-care provider about any necessary adjustments to their exercise routines during pregnancy and after giving birth.
- **For adults with chronic health conditions or disabilities**. These individuals should aim for 150–300 minutes of moderate-intensity exercise per week, or 75–150 minutes of vigorous-intensity exercise per week, if possible. Muscle-strengthening exercises involving all major muscle groups should also be done at least twice a week. If health issues prevent them from doing this much exercise, they should be as physically active as possible.

Fitness for Bone Disorders

- **For children and teens.**
  - Young children (ages three to five) should be physically active throughout the day. Adults should encourage them to engage in a variety of activities during play.
  - Children and teens (ages 6–17) should exercise for at least one hour every day, with most of it being moderate or vigorous intensity. They should also incorporate muscle-strengthening exercises at least three days a week and bone-strengthening exercises at least three days a week.[1]

Section 39.3 | Managing Osteogenesis Imperfecta

WHAT IS OSTEOGENESIS IMPERFECTA?

Osteogenesis imperfecta (OI), commonly known as "brittle bone disease," is a genetic disorder that most physicians rarely encounter in their careers. It is estimated that 25,000–50,000 people in the United States have OI, with the disorder occurring in approximately 1 in every 12,000–15,000 births. OI affects males and females equally and is found across all races and ethnic groups.

TREATMENTS

Since there is no cure for OI, treatment focuses on minimizing fractures, surgically correcting deformities, reducing bone fragility by increasing bone density, minimizing pain, and maximizing mobility and independent function. Some prescribed treatments include the following:
- behavioral and lifestyle modifications to avoid situations that may cause a fracture
- rehabilitation, including water therapy and physical activity

---

[1] "Exercise for Your Bone Health," National Institute of Arthritis and Musculoskeletal and Skin Diseases (NIAMS), May 1, 2023. Available online. URL: www.niams.nih.gov/health-topics/exercise-your-bone-health. Accessed September 10, 2024.

- weight management
- orthopedic surgery

BEHAVIORAL AND LIFESTYLE MODIFICATIONS
- Proper techniques for standing, sitting, and lifting are essential to protect the spine.
- Activities that jar or twist the spine, such as jumping and games "like crack-the-whip," should be avoided.
- Modify the home and school environment as needed to accommodate short stature or low strength and to promote independent function.
- Maintain a safe environment. For young children, this includes keeping the floor free of obstacles that could cause accidents.
- Develop healthy lifestyle habits, including a balanced diet and exercise, to maximize peak bone mass, build muscle strength, and avoid obesity.

REHABILITATION, PHYSICAL THERAPY, OCCUPATIONAL THERAPY, AND PHYSICAL ACTIVITY
- Most children with OI benefit from physical activity programs.
- Treatment plans should promote and maintain optimal function, including early intervention, muscle strengthening, aerobic conditioning, and, when possible, protected ambulation.
- Infancy presents many opportunities to develop strength and avoid deformities such as torticollis, which are often seen in children with OI.
- Proper positioning is critical to prevent contracture and malformation. A child with OI should not remain in a fixed position, either lying down or sitting, for extended periods.
- Immobilization reduces lean muscle mass and cardiovascular fitness and causes bone density to decline rapidly.

Fitness for Bone Disorders

- Postfracture therapy is necessary to mitigate the effects of immobilization on bone density and strength.
- The goal of physical therapy should be to improve function, fitness, and independent movement.
- Exercise should be prescribed based on the specific strengths and needs of each child, with a focus on posture and stamina.
- Recreational activities can provide fun, socialization, and physical benefits to children with OI.
- Swimming and water therapy are highly recommended.

PSYCHOLOGICAL, EMOTIONAL, AND SOCIAL SUPPORT

- Coping with and adjusting to having a child with OI is stressful for families. The strain of having a baby with a serious medical condition can deplete family resources and may lead to postpartum depression in the mother. Families will need referrals to various medical specialists.
- At different times, families will also need referrals to social services and resource organizations within the community.
- Siblings of the affected child may also require support.
- Addressing issues related to self-esteem, sexuality, and peer integration is crucial for the overall well-being of the older child or teenager with OI.
- The mental health concerns of children with OI are similar to those of other children with chronic health conditions and may include the following:
  - depression
  - fear of an early death
  - fear of strangers
  - anxiety in crowds

TRANSITION TO ADULT CARE

- Like other older children and teens, individuals with OI need age-appropriate information about sexuality and childbearing.

- Information about the benefits of healthy lifestyle choices—such as avoiding smoking, abstaining from alcohol abuse, and maintaining a healthy weight—is as important for young people with OI as for their unaffected peers.[1]

---

[1] "Guide to Osteogenesis Imperfecta," National Institutes of Health (NIH), November 2007. Available online. URL: www.govinfo.gov/content/pkg/GOVPUB-HE20-PURL-LPS115586/pdf/GOVPUB-HE20-PURL-LPS115586.pdf. Accessed September 10, 2024.

Chapter 40 | Fitness for Asthma

PHYSICAL ACTIVITY AND ASTHMA MANAGEMENT
Regular physical activity is important to the health and well-being of all individuals. However, people with asthma and their families often view asthma as a barrier to physical activity. Asthma is a common but serious chronic disease that affects about 1 in 10 children and many adults. Poorly controlled asthma can lead to debilitating symptoms, work absences, and life-threatening events that require emergency care. Asthma can limit a person's ability to engage in daily activities, work, and sleep, all of which are critical to overall well-being.

When asthma is well managed and controlled, people with asthma should be able to participate fully in all activities, including vigorous exercise.

Asthma is a serious chronic lung disease that inflames and narrows the airways. Although inflammation is a helpful defense mechanism, it can be harmful if it occurs at the wrong time or persists longer than necessary. Ongoing inflammation (swelling) makes the airways in the lungs more sensitive to asthma "triggers," such as:
- bacteria
- viruses
- dust
- tobacco smoke
- strong odors

The immune system of a person with asthma overreacts to these triggers by releasing cells and chemicals that cause the following changes in the airways:
- the inner linings of the airways become inflamed (swollen), leaving less room for air to move through
- the muscles surrounding the airways tighten, narrowing the airways even more (bronchospasm)
- the mucus glands in the airways produce thick mucus, further blocking the airways

These changes can make breathing difficult and can cause:
- coughing
- wheezing
- chest tightness
- shortness of breath

If the inflammation associated with asthma is not treated, exposure to asthma triggers will increase the inflammation, leading to more frequent symptoms.

EXERCISE-INDUCED ASTHMA

Exercise-induced asthma (also called "exercise-induced bronchospasm") is asthma triggered by physical activity. Vigorous exercise can cause symptoms in individuals whose asthma is not well controlled. Some people may experience asthma symptoms only when they exercise.

Asthma varies from person to person and can change from season to season or even hour to hour. At times, physical activity programs may need to be temporarily modified, such as by adjusting the type, intensity, duration, or frequency of activity. However, people with asthma should be included in activities as much as possible. Being excluded from activities can lead to:
- feelings of isolation
- loss of self-esteem
- unnecessary restriction of activity
- poor physical fitness

ASTHMA MEDICATIONS

Many people with asthma require both long-term control medications and quick-relief medications. These medications prevent and treat symptoms, enabling individuals to participate safely and fully in physical activities.

- **Long-term control medications are usually taken daily to control underlying airway inflammation and prevent asthma symptoms**. These medications can significantly reduce the need for quick-relief medication. Inhaled corticosteroids are the most effective long-term control medications for asthma. It is important to remember that inhaled corticosteroids are generally safe for long-term use when taken as prescribed. They are not addictive and are different from illegal anabolic steroids used by some athletes to build muscles.
- **Quick-relief medications (also known as "short-acting bronchodilators") are taken as needed for rapid, short-term relief of asthma symptoms**. These medications help stop asthma attacks by temporarily relaxing the muscles around the airways, but they do not treat the underlying airway inflammation that caused the symptoms.

For those with exercise-induced asthma, health-care providers may recommend taking quick-relief medication five minutes before participating in physical activities to prevent symptoms.

MODIFYING PHYSICAL ACTIVITIES FOR ASTHMA

People who follow their asthma action plans and keep their asthma under control can usually participate in a full range of sports and physical activities. Activities that are more intense and sustained, such as long periods of running, basketball, and soccer, are more likely to provoke asthma symptoms. Nevertheless, most people diagnosed with asthma, including exercise-induced asthma, can participate in these activities if their asthma is properly treated. Olympic athletes with asthma have demonstrated that vigorous activities are possible with good asthma management.

Fitness and Exercise Sourcebook, Seventh Edition

When an individual experiences asthma symptoms or is recovering from a recent asthma attack, physical activities should be temporarily modified in type, length, and/or frequency to reduce the risk of further symptoms. Work with health-care providers and others to plan appropriate activities until full recovery.[1]

---

[1] "Asthma and Physical Activity in the School: Making a Difference," National Heart, Lung, and Blood Institute (NHLBI), April 2012. Available online. URL: www.nhlbi.nih.gov/sites/default/files/publications/12-3651.pdf. Accessed September 10, 2024.

Chapter 41 | Managing Diabetes through Physical Activity

HEALTHY LIVING TO MANAGE DIABETES
Healthy living may help maintain your blood pressure, cholesterol, and blood glucose (blood sugar) levels within the range recommended by your primary health-care professional, who may be a doctor, physician assistant, or nurse practitioner. It can also help prevent or delay diabetes-related complications that affect your heart, kidneys, eyes, brain, and other parts of your body.

Making lifestyle changes can be challenging, but starting with small steps and building from there can benefit your health. Consider seeking support from family, friends, and other trusted individuals in your community. Your health-care professionals can also provide helpful information.

HOW PHYSICAL ACTIVITY HELPS MANAGE DIABETES
Research shows that regular physical activity helps people manage diabetes and maintain overall health. The benefits of physical activity include:
- lower blood glucose, blood pressure, and cholesterol levels
- improved heart health
- healthier weight
- better mood and sleep
- improved balance and memory

Talk with your health-care professional before starting a new physical activity or modifying your routine. They can suggest activities based on your ability, schedule, meal plan, interests, and diabetes medications. Your health-care professional may also advise you on the best times of day to be active or how to manage your blood glucose levels during exercise.

TYPES OF PHYSICAL ACTIVITY FOR PEOPLE WITH DIABETES

People with diabetes can stay active, even if they take insulin or use technology such as insulin pumps.

It is beneficial to try different kinds of physical activities. While being more active may provide greater health benefits, any amount of physical activity is better than none. Start slowly with activities you enjoy, and gradually increase your level of effort over time. Having a friend or family member join you may help you stay motivated.

The types of activities you do may vary if you are 65 years or older, pregnant, or have a disability or health condition. Physical activities may also need to be adjusted for children and teens. Ask your health-care professional about activities that are safe for you.

Aerobic Activities

Aerobic activities make you breathe harder and raise your heart rate. You can try walking, dancing, swimming, or wheelchair rolling. Most adults should aim for at least 150 minutes of moderate-intensity physical activity per week, which breaks down to about 30 minutes per day on most days. You can split the 30 minutes into smaller increments throughout the day and still gain the benefits.

Strength Training or Resistance Training

Strength training or resistance training helps strengthen muscles and bones. You can try lifting weights or doing exercises such as wall pushups or arm raises. Aim to do this type of training twice a week.

Balance and Stretching Activities

Balance and stretching activities improve flexibility, mobility, and strength. Examples include standing on one leg or stretching your

Managing Diabetes through Physical Activity

legs while sitting on the floor. Try to engage in these activities two or three times a week.

Some balance-related activities may be unsafe for individuals with nerve damage or vision problems caused by diabetes. Consult your health-care professional for advice on safe activities.

STAY SAFE DURING PHYSICAL ACTIVITY
Staying safe during physical activity is important. Here are some tips to keep in mind:
- **Drink liquids**. Staying hydrated helps prevent dehydration. Water is the best option for hydration, while sports drinks may contain unnecessary sugars and calories for most moderate activities.
- **Avoid low blood glucose**. Check your blood glucose levels before, during, and after physical activity. Physical activity can lower your blood glucose levels, and this effect may last for hours or even days. Those who take insulin or certain diabetes medications, such as sulfonylureas, are more likely to experience low blood glucose. Ask your health-care professional if you should adjust your insulin dose or eat carbohydrates before, during, or after physical activity. Low blood glucose is a medical emergency and should be treated immediately. Learn how to treat low blood glucose and consider wearing a medical alert bracelet.
- **Avoid high blood glucose and ketoacidosis**. Reducing insulin before exercise may help prevent low blood glucose but may increase the risk of high blood glucose. When the body cannot use glucose for energy, it uses fat instead, leading to the production of ketones. High levels of ketones in the blood can result in diabetic ketoacidosis (DKA), a medical emergency. DKA is more common in people with type 1 diabetes, but it can also affect individuals with type 2 diabetes who have lost the ability to produce insulin. Ask your health-care professional about how much insulin to take before

exercise, whether to test for ketones, and what level of ketones is dangerous for you.
- **Take care of your feet**. Diabetes can cause foot problems due to nerve and blood vessel damage. Wear comfortable, supportive shoes and take care of your feet before, during, and after physical activity to prevent issues.[1]

---

[1] "Healthy Living with Diabetes," National Institute of Diabetes and Digestive and Kidney Diseases (NIDDK), October 2023. Available online. URL: www.niddk.nih.gov/health-information/diabetes/overview/diet-eating-physical-activity. Accessed September 10, 2024.

Chapter 42 | Physical Activity and Cancer

PHYSICAL ACTIVITY AND SEDENTARY BEHAVIOR

Physical activity is defined as any movement that uses skeletal muscles and requires more energy than resting. Examples of physical activity include walking, running, dancing, biking, swimming, performing household chores, exercising, and engaging in sports activities.

A measure called the "metabolic equivalent of task" (MET) is used to characterize the intensity of physical activity. One MET represents the rate of energy expended by a person sitting at rest. Light-intensity activities expend fewer than three METs, moderate-intensity activities expend three to six METs, and vigorous activities expend six or more METs.

Sedentary behavior refers to any waking activity characterized by an energy expenditure of 1.5 or fewer METs while sitting, reclining, or lying down. Examples of sedentary behaviors include most office work, driving a vehicle, and sitting while watching television.

A person can be physically active and still spend a significant amount of time being sedentary.

THE LINK BETWEEN PHYSICAL ACTIVITY AND REDUCED CANCER RISK

Evidence linking higher physical activity to lower cancer risk primarily comes from observational studies, in which individuals report their physical activity and are followed for years for cancer diagnoses. Although observational studies cannot prove a causal relationship, similar results across different populations and a potential mechanism for a causal relationship provide evidence of a causal connection.

There is strong evidence that higher levels of physical activity are associated with a lower risk of several types of cancer:

- **Bladder cancer.** A 2014 meta-analysis of 11 cohort studies and 4 case-control studies found that the risk of bladder cancer was 15 percent lower for individuals with the highest levels of recreational or occupational physical activity compared to those with the lowest levels. A pooled analysis of over 1 million individuals found that leisure-time physical activity was associated with a 13 percent reduced risk of bladder cancer.
- **Breast cancer.** Many studies have shown that physically active women have a lower risk of breast cancer than inactive women. A 2016 meta-analysis of 38 cohort studies found that the most physically active women had a 12–21 percent lower risk of breast cancer than the least physically active women. The reductions in risk are similar for both premenopausal and postmenopausal women. Women who increase their physical activity after menopause may also have a lower risk of breast cancer.
- **Colon cancer.** A 2016 meta-analysis of 126 studies found that individuals who engaged in the highest levels of physical activity had a 19 percent lower risk of colon cancer than those who were the least physically active.
- **Endometrial cancer.** Several meta-analyses and cohort studies have examined the relationship between physical activity and the risk of endometrial cancer. A meta-analysis of 33 studies found that highly physically active women had a 20 percent lower risk of endometrial cancer than women with low levels of physical activity. Some evidence suggests that the association may be indirect, with physical activity reducing obesity, a strong risk factor for endometrial cancer.

- **Esophageal cancer.** A 2014 meta-analysis of 9 cohort and 15 case-control studies found that individuals who were most physically active had a 21 percent lower risk of esophageal adenocarcinoma than those who were least physically active.
- **Kidney (renal cell) cancer.** A 2013 meta-analysis of 11 cohort studies and 8 case-control studies found that the most physically active individuals had a 12 percent lower risk of renal cancer compared to the least active. A pooled analysis of over 1 million individuals linked leisure-time physical activity to a 23 percent reduced risk of kidney cancer.
- **Stomach (gastric) cancer.** A 2016 meta-analysis of 10 cohort studies and 12 case-control studies found that individuals who were the most physically active had a 19 percent lower risk of stomach cancer than those who were the least active.

There is also some evidence that physical activity may reduce the risk of lung cancer, although differences in smoking habits may account for this association. A 2016 meta-analysis of 25 observational studies found that physical activity was associated with a reduced risk of lung cancer in former and current smokers but not in never-smokers.

For several other cancers, the evidence of an association is more limited, including cancers of the blood, pancreas, prostate, ovaries, thyroid, liver, and rectum.

BIOLOGICAL EFFECTS OF EXERCISE ON CANCER RISK REDUCTION

Exercise has many biological effects on the body that may explain its associations with reduced cancer risks, including:
- lowering levels of sex hormones, such as estrogen, and growth factors that have been linked to cancer development and progression (breast, colon)
- preventing high blood insulin levels, which have been linked to cancer development and progression (breast, colon)

- reducing inflammation
- improving immune system function
- altering bile acid metabolism, reducing gastrointestinal exposure to suspected carcinogens (colon)
- reducing the time food spends in the digestive system, decreasing exposure to possible carcinogens (colon)
- helping prevent obesity, a risk factor for many cancers

THE EFFECT OF SEDENTARY BEHAVIOR ON CANCER RISK

Fewer studies have examined the relationship between sedentary behavior and cancer risk than physical activity and cancer risk. However, sedentary behavior—sitting, reclining, or lying down for extended periods (excluding sleep)—is a risk factor for many chronic conditions and premature death. It may also be associated with an increased risk of certain cancers.

PHYSICAL ACTIVITY RECOMMENDATIONS FOR CANCER RISK REDUCTION

The *Physical Activity Guidelines for Americans, 2nd edition*, released in 2018, recommends the following for substantial health benefits and to reduce the risk of chronic diseases, including cancer:

- 150–300 minutes of moderate-intensity aerobic activity, 75–100 minutes of vigorous-intensity aerobic activity, or an equivalent combination each week; this physical activity can be done in episodes of any length
- muscle-strengthening activities at least two days a week
- balance training, in addition to aerobic and muscle-strengthening activities

PHYSICAL ACTIVITY FOR CANCER SURVIVORS

The 2018 American College of Sports Medicine International Multidisciplinary Roundtable on Physical Activity and Cancer Prevention and Control concluded that exercise training and testing are generally safe for cancer survivors and that all survivors should maintain some level of physical activity.

Physical Activity and Cancer

The Roundtable found:
- strong evidence that moderate-intensity aerobic training and/or resistance exercise during and after cancer treatment can reduce anxiety, depressive symptoms, and fatigue, while improving health-related quality of life (QOL) and physical function
- strong evidence that exercise training is safe for individuals who have or might develop breast cancer-related lymphedema
- some evidence that exercise benefits bone health and sleep quality
- insufficient evidence that physical activity prevents cardiotoxicity or chemotherapy-induced peripheral neuropathy or improves cognitive function, falls, nausea, pain, sexual function, or treatment tolerance

Additionally, research has suggested that physical activity may benefit survival rates in patients with breast, colorectal, and prostate cancers:
- **Breast cancer.** A 2019 systematic review and meta-analysis found that breast cancer survivors who were the most physically active had a 42 percent lower risk of death from any cause and a 40 percent lower risk of death from breast cancer than the least physically active survivors.
- **Colorectal cancer.** Multiple epidemiologic studies suggest that physical activity after a colorectal cancer diagnosis is associated with a 30 percent lower risk of death from colorectal cancer and a 38 percent lower risk of death from any cause.
- **Prostate cancer.** Limited evidence suggests that physical activity after a prostate cancer diagnosis is associated with a 33 percent lower risk of death from prostate cancer and a 45 percent lower risk of death from any cause.

There is very limited evidence of physical activity's effects on survival for other cancers, including non-Hodgkin lymphoma, stomach cancer, and malignant glioma.[1]

---

[1] "Physical Activity and Cancer," National Cancer Institute (NCI), February 10, 2020. Available online. URL: www.cancer.gov/about-cancer/causes-prevention/risk/obesity/physical-activity-fact-sheet. Accessed September 10, 2024.

Chapter 43 | Overcoming the Challenges of an Inactive Lifestyle

WHAT IS AN INACTIVE LIFESTYLE?
Being a couch potato, not exercising, or living a sedentary or inactive lifestyle—these phrases all describe a lifestyle that involves a lot of sitting and lying down and little to no exercise.

In the United States and around the world, people are spending more time doing sedentary activities. During our leisure time, we often sit while using computers, watching TV, or playing video games. Many jobs are becoming more sedentary, with long hours spent sitting at a desk. Additionally, most of our daily transportation involves sitting in cars, on buses, or on trains.

HOW DOES AN INACTIVE LIFESTYLE AFFECT YOUR BODY?
An inactive lifestyle can have several negative effects on the body:
- Fewer calories are burned, increasing the likelihood of weight gain.
- Muscle strength and endurance may decrease due to lack of use.
- Bones may weaken and lose mineral content.
- Metabolism may slow, making it harder to break down fats and sugars.
- The immune system may become less effective.
- Blood circulation may worsen.
- Inflammation in the body may increase.
- Hormonal imbalances may develop.

Fitness and Exercise Sourcebook, Seventh Edition

WHAT ARE THE HEALTH RISKS OF AN INACTIVE LIFESTYLE?
An inactive lifestyle can contribute to many chronic diseases. Without regular exercise, the risks of the following conditions are higher:
- obesity
- heart diseases, including coronary artery disease and heart attack
- high blood pressure (HBP)
- high cholesterol
- stroke
- metabolic syndrome
- type 2 diabetes
- certain cancers, including colon, breast, and uterine cancers
- osteoporosis and falls
- increased feelings of depression and anxiety

A sedentary lifestyle can also increase the risk of premature death. The more sedentary you are, the higher your health risks become.

HOW CAN YOU GET STARTED WITH EXERCISE?
If you have been inactive, it is important to start slowly and gradually increase your exercise. Any amount of exercise is better than none. The goal is to eventually meet the recommended amount of exercise for your age and health.

There are many ways to incorporate exercise into your life. It is important to find the types of physical activity that work best for you. You can also make small changes to increase activity at home and at work.

HOW CAN YOU BE MORE ACTIVE AROUND THE HOUSE?
Here are some ways to increase physical activity at home:
- **Housework, gardening, and yard work are all forms of physical activity.** To increase intensity, try doing them at a more vigorous pace.

Overcoming the Challenges of an Inactive Lifestyle

- **Keep moving while watching TV.** Lift hand weights, do gentle yoga stretches, or use an exercise bike. Instead of using the remote, get up to change the channels.
- **Work out at home using a workout video (on TV or the Internet).**
- **Go for a walk in your neighborhood.** Walking with your dog, your kids, or a friend can make it more enjoyable.
- **Stand up when talking on the phone.**
- **Consider getting exercise equipment for your home.** While treadmills and elliptical trainers can be expensive, yoga balls, exercise mats, stretch bands, and hand weights are more affordable options for working out at home.

HOW CAN YOU BE MORE ACTIVE AT WORK?

Most people sit while working, often in front of a computer. Less than 20 percent of Americans have physically active jobs. Here are some tips to help you stay active during a busy workday:

- Get up from your chair and move around at least once an hour.
- Stand while talking on the phone.
- Ask if your company can provide a stand-up or treadmill desk.
- Take the stairs instead of the elevator.
- Use your break or lunch hour to walk around the building.
- Walk to a colleague's office instead of sending an email.
- Hold "walking" or standing meetings with co-workers instead of sitting in a conference room.[1]

---

[1] MedlinePlus, "Health Risks of an Inactive Lifestyle," National Institutes of Health (NIH), September 1, 2017. Available online. URL: https://medlineplus.gov/healthrisksofaninactivelifestyle.html. Accessed September 10, 2024.

Chapter 44 | The Benefits of Quitting Smoking for Fitness and Health

WHY YOU SHOULD QUIT
There are many great reasons to stop smoking. Understand how smoking affects you and your loved ones, and explore the benefits of quitting. Reflect on why you want to be smoke-free and remind yourself of these reasons when you need extra motivation.

HOW SMOKING AFFECTS YOUR WORKOUT
When you smoke, you harm your ability to exercise and maintain physical fitness. Smoking affects your athletic performance in several ways.

Blood
The nicotine and carbon monoxide from smoking can make your blood "sticky," and your arteries may narrow. Narrow arteries reduce the flow of blood to your heart, muscles, and other organs, making exercise harder. During exercise, blood flow boosts the oxygen supply to your muscles. If your muscles do not get oxygen fast enough, your body cannot perform as well.

Heart
Smoking increases your resting heart rate, which is the number of beats per minute your heart produces when you are not active. Smoking raises this number because of the extra work your heart has to do to keep your body going. Your heart rate could potentially

Fitness and Exercise Sourcebook, Seventh Edition

rise to dangerous levels when you engage in physical activities. A higher-than-normal resting heart rate increases the risk of death.

Lungs

You are able to exercise better when your lung capacity is strong, and your lungs function well. Smoking decreases lung capacity. The tar in cigarette smoke coats your lungs and reduces the elasticity of the air sacs. Smoking also produces phlegm, which can make your lungs congested. Even smoking a few cigarettes a day can decrease your body's ability to use oxygen effectively.

USE EXERCISE TO HELP YOU QUIT

Exercise can be an important part of your plan to quit smoking. It reduces cravings and helps you manage withdrawal symptoms and stress. Plus, when you quit, your heart rate will decrease, your blood circulation will improve, and your lung function will recover—leading to better workout performance.[1]

Fight Cravings with Exercise

Cravings for a cigarette are one of the most common symptoms of nicotine withdrawal when quitting smoking. It helps to have a plan to manage cravings when they strike. Including exercise in the plan can assist in overcoming cravings.

Exercise serves as a distraction and keeps the body occupied until the craving passes.

Exercise also has additional benefits:
- Studies show that even short periods of physical activity, especially aerobic exercise, reduce the urge to smoke. Aerobic exercise is any physical activity that causes sweating, heavier breathing, and a faster heart rate. It strengthens the heart and lungs. Examples include walking, swimming, running, dancing, cycling, and boxing.

---

[1] Smokefree.gov, "How Smoking Affects Your Workout," U.S. Department of Health and Human Services (HHS), September 8, 2016. Available online. URL: https://smokefree.gov/quit-smoking/why-you-should-quit/how-smoking-affects-your-workout. Accessed September 11, 2024.

The Benefits of Quitting Smoking for Fitness and Health

- Withdrawal symptoms and cravings for cigarettes decrease during exercise and up to 50 minutes after exercising.
- Exercise reduces appetite and helps limit the weight gain that some people experience when quitting smoking.
- Exercise assists in managing stress and boosts energy levels.
- Exercise can enhance mood. When feeling down, activities such as walking, jumping rope, or running up and down stairs can lift one's mood.

Get Physical

Here are some tips to start exercising and manage cravings effectively:

- **Set aside a regular time for exercise that fits into the schedule.**
- **Aim for 30 minutes of physical activity on most days of the week.** If 30 minutes is not available, studies show that exercising for 10 minutes three times a day offers the same benefits as 30 minutes of continuous exercise.
- **Choose enjoyable activities.** Walking is a simple way to increase physical activity. Other options might include biking, swimming, dancing, or yoga. Even housework or gardening can offer exercise benefits. Playing music while cleaning can help increase the pace.
- **Incorporate exercise into daily routines.** Take the stairs instead of the elevator, or use the stairs instead of an escalator at the mall. Park farther away and walk to the destination.
- **Plan physical activities with family, friends, or co-workers, such as a hike or a volleyball game.**
- **Change the exercise routine or try new activities occasionally to avoid boredom.**[2]

---

[2] Smokefree.gov, "Fight Cravings with Exercise," U.S. Department of Health and Human Services (HHS), September 8, 2016. Available online. URL: https://smokefree.gov/challenges-when-quitting/cravings-triggers/fight-cravings-exercise. Accessed September 11, 2024.

Chapter 45 | The Importance of Quality Sleep for Well-Being

WHAT ARE SLEEP DEPRIVATION AND DEFICIENCY?
Sleep deprivation occurs when you do not get enough sleep. Sleep deficiency is a broader concept and occurs if you experience one or more of the following:
- You do not get enough sleep (sleep deprivation).
- You sleep at the wrong time of day.
- You do not sleep well or fail to get the different types of sleep your body needs.
- You have a sleep disorder that prevents you from getting enough sleep or causes poor-quality sleep.

Sleeping is a basic human need, such as eating, drinking, and breathing. Like these other needs, sleep is vital for good health and well-being throughout one's lifetime.

According to the Centers for Disease Control and Prevention (CDC), about one in three adults in the United States report not getting enough rest or sleep every day. Nearly 40 percent of adults report falling asleep during the day without meaning to at least once a month. Additionally, an estimated 50–70 million Americans have chronic or ongoing sleep disorders.

HOW SLEEP AFFECTS YOUR HEALTH
Getting enough quality sleep at the right times can help protect your mental health, physical health, quality of life (QOL), and safety.

How Do I Know If I Am Not Getting Enough Sleep?
Sleep deficiency may cause you to feel tired during the day, and you may not feel refreshed or alert when you wake up. Sleep deficiency can interfere with work, school, driving, and social functioning.

You may be sleep deficient if you often feel like you could doze off while:
- sitting and reading or watching TV
- sitting still in a public place, such as a movie theater, meeting, or classroom
- riding in a car for an hour without stopping
- sitting and talking to someone
- sitting quietly after lunch
- sitting in traffic for a few minutes

Sleep deficiency can cause problems with learning, focusing, and reacting. You may have difficulty making decisions, solving problems, remembering things, managing emotions and behavior, and coping with change. Tasks may take longer to complete, and your reaction time may slow, leading to mistakes.

Symptoms in Children
The symptoms of sleep deficiency may differ between children and adults. Sleep-deficient children might be overly active and have trouble paying attention. They may misbehave, and their school performance may suffer.

Sleep-deficient children may feel angry and impulsive and experience mood swings, sadness, or depression. They may also lack motivation.

SLEEP AND YOUR HEALTH
The way you feel while you are awake depends partly on what happens while you sleep. During sleep, your body is working to support healthy brain function and maintain your physical health. In children and teens, sleep also helps support growth and development.

The damage caused by sleep deficiency can occur suddenly, such as during a car crash, or it can harm you over time. For example, ongoing sleep deficiency can increase your risk of chronic health problems. It can also affect how well you think, react, work, learn, and interact with others.

Mental Health Benefits

Sleep helps your brain work properly. While you sleep, your brain is preparing for the next day. It forms new pathways to help you learn and remember information.

Studies show that a good night's sleep improves learning and problem-solving skills. Sleep also helps you focus, make decisions, and be creative.

Sleep deficiency, on the other hand, alters brain activity. If you are sleep deficient, you may have difficulty making decisions, solving problems, controlling emotions and behavior, and coping with change. Sleep deficiency is also linked to depression, suicide, and risk-taking behaviors.

Children and teens who are sleep deficient may have difficulty getting along with others. They may feel angry and impulsive, experience mood swings, feel sad or depressed, or lack motivation. These children may also struggle to pay attention, get lower grades, and feel stressed.

Physical Health Benefits

Sleep plays a critical role in your physical health.

Good-quality sleep offers numerous health benefits, including the following:

- **Heals and repairs your heart and blood vessels**.
- **Helps maintain a healthy balance of hormones that control hunger (ghrelin) and fullness (leptin)**. When you do not get enough sleep, your ghrelin levels increase, and your leptin levels decrease, making you feel hungrier than when you are well-rested.
- **Affects how your body reacts to insulin, the hormone that controls blood glucose (sugar) levels**. Sleep deficiency results in higher-than-normal blood sugar levels, which may increase your risk of diabetes.
- **Supports healthy growth and development**. Deep sleep triggers the release of a hormone that promotes normal

growth in children and teens. This hormone also boosts muscle mass and helps repair cells and tissues in children, teens, and adults. Sleep also plays a role in puberty and fertility.
- **Enhances your body's ability to fight germs and illness.** Ongoing sleep deficiency may alter your immune response, making it harder for your body to fight common infections.
- **Reduces your risk of health problems such as heart disease, high blood pressure (HBP), obesity, and stroke.**

HEALTHY SLEEP HABITS

You can take steps to improve your sleep habits. First, make sure you give yourself enough time to sleep. With adequate sleep each night, you may find that you feel happier and more productive during the day.

Sleep is often the first thing busy people cut from their schedules. Prioritizing sleep is important for protecting your health and well-being now and in the future.

To improve your sleep habits, you can adopt several practices, including the following:
- **Go to bed and wake up at the same time every day.** Establish a set bedtime and bedtime routine for children. Avoid using the child's bedroom for timeouts or punishment.
- **Try to maintain the same sleep schedule on weeknights and weekends.** Keep the difference to no more than an hour. Staying up late and sleeping in on weekends can disrupt your body clock's sleep-wake rhythm.
- **Use the hour before bed for quiet time.** Avoid intense exercise and bright artificial light, such as from a TV or computer screen. The light may signal the brain that it is time to be awake.
- **Avoid heavy or large meals within a few hours of bedtime.** A light snack is acceptable. Also, avoid consuming alcohol before bed.

- **Avoid nicotine (such as cigarettes) and caffeine (found in caffeinated sodas, coffee, tea, and chocolate).** Both substances are stimulants and can interfere with sleep. The effects of caffeine can last up to eight hours, so a cup of coffee in the late afternoon may make it difficult to fall asleep at night.
- **Spend time outside every day, if possible, and engage in physical activity.**
- **Keep your bedroom quiet, cool, and dark.** A dim night light is acceptable if necessary.
- **Take a hot bath or practice relaxation techniques before bed.**
- **Napping during the day may boost alertness and performance.** However, if you have trouble falling asleep at night, limit naps or take them earlier in the afternoon. Adults should nap for no more than 20 minutes.

HOW IS SLEEP DEPRIVATION TREATED?

If your doctor diagnoses you with a sleep disorder, they may discuss healthy sleep habits with you. Your treatment options will depend on the type of sleep disorder you have.
- For sleep apnea, the goal of treatment is to keep your airways open during sleep. Treatment may include using a continuous positive airway pressure (CPAP) machine, other breathing devices, therapy, or surgery.
- For narcolepsy and insomnia, treatment options may include medications and behavioral changes.[1]

---

[1] "What Are Sleep Deprivation and Deficiency?" National Heart, Lung, and Blood Institute (NHLBI), March 24, 2022. Available online. URL: www.nhlbi.nih.gov/health/sleep-deprivation. Accessed September 11, 2024.

Part 7 | Health and Wellness Trends

Chapter 46 | Top Fitness Trends of 2023

The National Institutes of Health (NIH) Health and Wellness Council's 2023 Top Fitness Trends highlight emerging fitness approaches, including wearable technology, body weight training, and strength training. Outdoor activities and fitness programs for older adults reflect a growing focus on personalized, accessible health solutions.

WEARABLE TECHNOLOGY
Wearable technology ranges from smartwatches to necklaces, as well as clips for the hip and shoe, and even rings. These devices automatically track metrics such as calories burned, steps taken, and distance traveled. Some monitors allow users to create challenges or competitions with friends, which can motivate some individuals.

Wearable technology encourages self-monitoring, a powerful behavior change tool that has been shown to be an effective strategy for achieving health goals such as weight loss.

STRENGTH TRAINING WITH FREE WEIGHTS
Free weights are a form of strength training that involves resistance exercises using "free" objects that are not attached to anything and can be picked up and moved. These include:
- medicine balls
- barbells
- dumbbells
- kettlebells
- sandbags

Fitness and Exercise Sourcebook, Seventh Edition

- resistance bands
- sand bells

BODY WEIGHT TRAINING

Body weight training programs utilize the body's weight as the training modality through variable resistance and neuromotor movements across multiple planes. Since body weight training requires little to no equipment, it is an inexpensive and functional way to exercise effectively.

FUNCTIONAL FITNESS TRAINING

Functional fitness training is a trend that uses strength training and other movements to improve balance, coordination, strength, and endurance. The goal is to enhance the ability to perform activities of daily living.

FITNESS PROGRAMS FOR OLDER ADULTS

People today are living longer, working longer, and staying healthy and active much longer than previous generations. Fitness programs for older adults cater specifically to the Baby Boomer and older generations, addressing their unique needs.

OUTDOOR ACTIVITIES

Perhaps due to the coronavirus 2019 (COVID-19) pandemic, outdoor activities such as small group walks, group rides, or organized hiking groups have gained popularity. These activities can range from short events to day- or week-long excursions. Participants typically meet in local parks, hiking areas, or bike trails with a designated leader.

Whether through wearable technology, strength training, or outdoor activities, these trends offer diverse ways for individuals to stay active and maintain a healthy lifestyle across different age groups.[1]

---

[1] Division of Occupational Health and Safety (DOHS), "NIH Health and Wellness Council Presents 2023 Top Fitness Trends," National Institutes of Health (NIH), February 15, 2023. Available online. URL: https://wellnessatnih.ors.od.nih.gov/news/Pages/NIH-Health-and-Wellness-Council-Presents-2023-Top-Fitness-Trends.aspx. Accessed September 11, 2024.

Chapter 47 | Wellness Tourism

THE EVOLUTION AND GROWTH OF WELLNESS TOURISM

The global wellness industry is a thriving and fast-growing sector, and one of its healthiest components is wellness tourism. The industry is currently valued at nearly $700 billion, with an annual growth rate expected to be close to 7.5 percent. Wellness tourists are considered high-value tourists, recognizing the benefit of paying for activities that promote their sense of well-being.

The concept of wellness and wellness-related activities has existed as long as human beings have, and like many things in our collective history, it has ebbed and flowed with prevailing circumstances. In more recent memory, the late 1980s and 1990s saw a surge in outward and aesthetics-driven wellness activities, largely in reaction to the obesity surge that began in the 1970s with the rise of fast food and "convenient" lifestyle.

On the fringes of this wellness wave were individuals already thinking differently. Although still motivated in part by outward aesthetics, they also looked inward, believing that inner wellness could lead to outer beauty. These ideas created the current wellness movement, emphasizing yoga, meditation, natural living, a connection to nature, avoidance of modern medicines, rediscovering the roots of food, and the birth of an "organic" life untouched by man-made chemicals. For a couple of decades, this remained a fringe movement. Then came the new millennium, and the Y2K bug heightened awareness of our reliance on technology. The Internet spread rapidly, introducing an array of products and services designed to make our lives more convenient, nearly ensuring we would never need to leave our desks. Being constantly connected became desirable, as did the latest gadgets, with the promise of rapid financial success through digital scaling seemingly within everyone's reach.

Within less than a decade, the corporate landscape transformed, with web-based companies dominating the stock market. The digital bubble burst in the early 2000s but was quickly forgotten, and continuous rapid growth became a corporate expectation.

The side effects of this fast-paced life, driven by technology and financial insecurity, began to take a toll on physical and mental health. This insecurity, coupled with digital exhaustion and the stress of making ends meet, gave birth to a new wave of wellness pursuits.

Today, wellness is defined as the pursuit of activities, products, and services that help individuals achieve physical, emotional, intellectual, spiritual, social, financial, and environmental well-being. Wellness is now a holistic concept, underlined by mindfulness—a more attentive way of living that considers the effect of individuals on their surroundings and vice versa, recognizing their interdependence.

In this context, wellness tourism is a natural byproduct of this evolution. For those practicing a mindful approach to living, wellness does not end at the airport check-in counter. Enabled by the ease and affordability of travel and global curiosity, the tourism industry has surged, accompanied by wellness-minded travelers.

Whether for the sole pursuit of wellness or as part of maintaining a mindful lifestyle, wellness tourism is on the rise, delivering travelers willing to invest in activities, products, and services they view as an investment in themselves.

KEY CHARACTERISTICS OF WELLNESS SEEKERS

- Self-development and continuous growth are points of pride and represent new milestones of success.
- Money spent on wellness is viewed as an investment in oneself—a secure investment in a world with little other means of security.
- Giving is more rewarding than getting.
- Being inspired and inspiring others is priceless and a strong driver of positive change.

Wellness Tourism

KEY GLOBAL TRENDS IN WELLNESS AND WELLNESS TOURISM
Nongeneric Wellness
- customized meditation (meditation tailored for specific effects, such as relaxation, energy, focus, or creativity)
- individualized self-development through learning and participation opportunities

Intimacy with Food
- mindful eating
- food as a human and cultural ritual
- food as a social connector
- food as a sensorial experience beyond just taste

Nature as Medicine
- prescribing time in nature as medicine is prescribed
- travel itineraries including time away from urban spaces to experience nature

Itineraries including Active Recovery
- recovery viewed as an active rather than a passive state
- more frequent active rest periods instead of fewer long ones
- utilizing therapies for low-cost, frequent active recovery, including:
  - cryotherapy
  - pulse electromagnetic field therapy
  - flotation therapy
  - sleeping pods
  - breathing pods
  - energy lounges
  - music therapy
  - art therapy
  - natural therapies
  - water massage
  - lymphatic bed massage
  - solariums for natural light exposure

THE RAPID GROWTH AND HIGH VALUE OF THE WELLNESS TOURISM INDUSTRY

The global wellness tourism industry has been a resounding success. A healthy 6.5 percent year-on-year growth has pushed global earnings to over half a trillion dollars, and this growth is expected to accelerate to 7.5 percent, bringing the industry close to a trillion dollars within the next three years.

The Global Wellness Institute divides wellness travelers into two types:

- **Primary wellness travelers**. Those are mainly motivated by wellness when choosing a destination or trip. These account for 11 percent of the total industry.
- **Secondary wellness travelers**. Those who seek to maintain wellness or engage in wellness activities during travel. These account for 89 percent of the total industry, highlighting the fact that wellness is no longer a niche subset of travelers.

Notably, international wellness travelers tend to outspend their counterparts by 53 percent on average, while domestic wellness tourists outspend theirs by 178 percent, making both groups high-value travelers.

While the industry is primarily driven by Western tourists and destinations, all markets are experiencing exponential growth, with the Asia-Pacific, the Middle East, Africa, and Latin America rapidly scaling up. The Middle East is second only to North America in terms of per capita expenditure on wellness tourism.[1]

---

[1] "Wellness Is in Our Nature: An Assessment of Jordan's Wellness Tourism Potential," U.S. Agency for International Development (USAID), June 2019. Available online. URL: https://pdf.usaid.gov/pdf_docs/PA00WPH2.pdf. Accessed September 11, 2024.

Chapter 48 | Smart Devices for Better Health Monitoring

With the increasing prevalence of smartwatches and fitness trackers, how can we harness the potential of these devices? A team of National Institutes of Health (NIH)-funded researchers has an idea: to use wearable sensors as a way to predict clinical test results, potentially serving as an early warning signal for underlying health issues.

"Consumer wearable devices have enormous untapped potential to facilitate the monitoring—and potentially, the prediction—of human health and disease," said Grace Peng, PhD, director of the National Institute of Biomedical Imaging and Bioengineering (NIBIB) program in Mathematical Modeling, Simulation, and Analysis. "This study, which investigates how data from smartwatches are associated with clinical laboratory tests, is an important step forward in this burgeoning field."

WHAT DID THE RESEARCHERS DO?

To explore how smartwatches could be incorporated into routine health care, the researchers evaluated how data from wearable devices compared with measurements taken in a clinical setting. They followed 54 participants for roughly three years. During this period, participants had about 40 clinic visits and wore a smartwatch for approximately 340 days. The smartwatch tracked four vital signs: heart rate, skin temperature, step count, and electrodermal activity (a measure of skin conductance). At the clinic, heart rate and oral temperature were measured, and clinical lab tests, including a complete blood count, a comprehensive metabolic panel, and a cholesterol panel, were conducted.

The researchers compared the vital sign data measured at clinic visits with continuous measurements from the smartwatch. They found that temperature readings were more consistent in the clinic, as oral temperature varied less than skin temperature measured by the wearable. However, heart rate measurements from the smartwatch were more accurate, as clinical heart rate readings had significantly more variability. "In a doctor's office, many variables can affect heart rate measurements, such as time of day, pre-appointment activities, or even nervousness," explained senior study author Michael Snyder, PhD, chair of the Department of Genetics at Stanford University School of Medicine. "Since a smartwatch is worn continuously, it provides a much more consistent heart rate measurement with less variability."

PREDICTING CLINICAL TEST RESULTS USING WEARABLE DATA

Next, the researchers sought to determine if smartwatch data could predict clinical lab test results. Using data gathered during the extended monitoring period, they analyzed over 150 features from the measurements, such as average heart rate during exercise, overnight variability in skin temperature, and overall electrodermal activity. They used machine learning models to combine these features and predict clinical lab results.

The predicted results were compared with actual lab test results from the clinic. The predictions aligned well with several clinical tests, with the most predictable results being for red blood cell (RBC) count, absolute monocyte count, hemoglobin (HBG) levels, and hematocrit (HCT) levels. Notably, electrodermal activity was a key factor in predicting RBC, HBG, and HCT test results.

"Electrodermal activity is typically measured in lie detector tests and is not part of standard clinical measurements," explained first author Jessilyn Dunn, PhD, assistant professor of biomedical engineering at Duke University. "It measures the opening of sweat glands, which can respond to stress, temperature, emotional state, or hydration. This technology could have significant clinical potential, such as detecting dehydration, especially in older individuals."

Other smartwatch data were important for predicting specific blood test results. For example, step count and skin temperature were key for predicting absolute monocyte count, while heart rate measurements were essential for predicting platelet count. The prediction of fasting plasma glucose relied on a combination of skin temperature, heart rate, and step count.

"Our results suggest that different physiological features are associated with the prediction of distinct clinical measurements," noted Dunn.

SMARTWATCHES AS EARLY WARNING SYSTEMS

The researchers emphasized that smartwatch data is not a replacement for clinical tests but could serve as an early warning system, prompting the wearer to consult their physician. "The power of wearable devices lies in their ability to detect changes from baseline readings," said Snyder. Even if some specific measurements are not highly accurate, the ability to detect shifts in vital signs could be extremely useful. "The current medical paradigm focuses on treating patients after they're already sick, not on monitoring healthy people for early disease detection," Snyder added. "We believe that data from smartwatches could help intercept emerging illnesses, potentially preventing more severe disease."[1]

---

[1] "Smartwatch Data Used to Predict Clinical Test Results," National Institute of Biomedical Imaging and Bioengineering (NIBIB), November 30, 2021. Available online. URL: www.nibib.nih.gov/news-events/newsroom/smartwatch-data-used-predict-clinical-test-results-4. Accessed September 11, 2024.

Chapter 49 | Improving Wellness Care through Technology

THE ROLE OF HEALTH INFORMATION TECHNOLOGIES

Smartphones and wearable devices such as fitness trackers offer a window into health and wellness by counting steps, monitoring sleep quality, and even measuring body temperature, blood oxygen levels, and heart rate. These technologies, which collect biological, behavioral, and environmental data, have become integrated into daily life for many people.

Although this reality might seem daunting—especially after watching one too many technological dystopian dramas—Dr. Sherine El-Toukhy's lab views these "health information technologies" as valuable tools that could help make the future of health care more equitable.

"Information technologies have been championed as a solution to some of the inefficiencies in health care," says Dr. El-Toukhy, an Earl Stadtman Investigator and National Institutes of Health (NIH) Distinguished Scholar at the National Institute on Minority Health and Health Disparities (NIMHD).

IMPROVING ACCESS FOR UNDERSERVED POPULATIONS

Because these devices can transmit data in real time, they have the potential to provide immediate health-care access, especially for traditionally underserved populations facing limited resources or living in remote areas. For individuals who might not otherwise have the means to communicate with a specialist, these technologies offer a way to share health and wellness metrics consistently and instantly, even if the provider is several states away. Smart devices could also alert the nearest hospital in the event of an emergency.

"Health information technology affords us the chance to improve our health-care system in several aspects, including effectiveness, timeliness, and efficiency," says Dr. El-Toukhy.

FACILITATING COMMUNICATION THROUGH DIGITAL TOOLS

Beyond improving communication from patient to physician, these technologies could also facilitate the flow of information from health-care systems to individuals. This was the focus of one of Dr. El-Toukhy's studies, where she and her collaborators set up an automatic referral system for hospital patients who identified as smokers or who consumed alcohol in excess. The system directed patients to two digital intervention apps, and researchers observed whether proactive electronic outreach encouraged more people to try them. Preliminary data suggests that about 15 percent of participants followed the referral to engage with the apps, demonstrating how health-care systems can connect patients with useful resources and potentially modify health behaviors.

"I think the best way for us as researchers is to really partner with entities that already have something in place that we can leverage," says Dr. El-Toukhy.

ADDRESSING BARRIERS TO DIGITAL HEALTH CARE

When imagining the future of information technologies built on personal data, concerns about privacy naturally arise. However, Dr. El-Toukhy has found that privacy is not the biggest barrier to recruiting participants, even among minority groups. She addresses concerns by being transparent and treating participants as partners, not just subjects.

"You can't be a parachute researcher—going in, taking the information you need, and then leaving," she explains. "You have to tell people what the research is for and how it's going to benefit them."

More pressing, according to Dr. El-Toukhy, is the potential of digital technologies to widen existing disparities. While virtual health

Improving Wellness Care through Technology

care can provide greater access for disadvantaged populations, it can also leave behind those without Internet access or the skills to navigate videoconferencing platforms. This concern became evident during the coronavirus 2019 (COVID-19) pandemic: telehealth visits increased by 50 percent in the first quarter of 2020 compared to the same period in 2019, according to the U.S. Centers for Disease Control and Prevention (CDC). However, the technological transition may exclude individuals who lack Internet access.

"You have to make sure things are as accessible to somebody who only has a middle school education as they are to someone who has a Ph.D.," she says. "We have to make sure that we're not leaving anyone behind."[1]

---

[1] "Smart Devices for Better Health," National Institutes of Health (NIH), May 24, 2023. Available online. URL: https://irp.nih.gov/our-research/research-in-action/smart-devices-for-better-health. Accessed September 11, 2024.

Part 8 | Additional Help and Information

Chapter 50 | Glossary of Terms Related to Fitness and Exercise

absolute intensity: The amount of energy used by the body per minute of activity.

aerobic exercise: Any continuous activity of large muscle groups that forces your heart and lungs to work harder. Aerobic means your heart and lungs are using oxygen.

aerobic physical activity: Aerobic (or endurance) physical activities use large muscle groups (back, chest, and legs) to increase heart rate and breathing for an extended period of time.

arthritis: A term used to describe more than 100 rheumatic diseases and conditions that affect joints, the tissues which surround the joint and other connective tissue.

balance: A performance-related component of physical fitness that involves the maintenance of the body's equilibrium while stationary or moving.

balance training: Static and dynamic exercises that are designed to improve individuals' ability to withstand challenges from postural sway or destabilizing stimuli caused by self-motion, the environment, or other objects.

body composition: A health-related component of physical fitness that applies to body weight and the relative amounts of muscle, fat, bone, and other vital tissues of the body. Most often, the components are limited to fat and lean body mass (or fat-free mass).

This glossary contains terms excerpted from documents produced by several sources deemed reliable.

body mass index (BMI): A measure of body weight relative to height. BMI is a tool that is often used to determine if a person is at a healthy weight, overweight, or obese, and whether a person's health is at risk due to his or her weight.

bone-strengthening activity: Physical activity primarily designed to increase the strength of specific sites in bones that make up the skeletal system.

calcium: A mineral that is an essential nutrient for bone health. It is also needed for the heart, muscles, and nerves to function properly and for blood to clot.

calisthenics: Physical exercises done without equipment to build muscular strength, endurance, and flexibility.

calorie: A unit of energy in food. Carbohydrates, fats, protein, and alcohol in the foods and drinks we eat provide food energy or "calories."

carbohydrate: A major source of energy in the diet. There are two kinds of carbohydrates—simple carbohydrates and complex carbohydrates: simple carbohydrates are sugars and complex carbohydrates include both starches and fiber.

cholesterol: A fatty substance present in all parts of the body. It is a component of cell membranes and is used to make vitamin D and some hormones. Some cholesterol in the body is produced by the liver and some is derived from food, particularly animal products.

cool down: A gradual reduction of the intensity of physical activity to allow physiological processes to return to normal.

corticosteroids: Steroid-type hormones that have antitumor activity in lymphomas and lymphoid leukemias. In addition, corticosteroids may be used for hormone replacement and for the management of some of the complications of cancer and its treatment.

dehydration: Excessive loss of body water that the body needs to carry on normal functions at an optimal level.

diet: What a person eats and drinks. Any type of eating plan.

duration: The length of time in which an activity or exercise is performed. Duration is generally expressed in minutes.

energy expenditure: The amount of energy that you use measured in calories. You use calories to breathe, send blood through your blood vessels, digest food, maintain posture, and be physically active.

exercise: A type of physical activity that involves planned, structured, and repetitive bodily movement done to maintain or improve one or more components of physical fitness.

Glossary of Terms Related to Fitness and Exercise

fat: A major source of energy in the diet. All food fats have nine calories per gram. Fat helps the body absorb fat-soluble vitamins, such as vitamins A, D, E, and K, and carotenoids.

flexibility: A health- and performance-related component of physical fitness that is the range of motion possible at a joint. Flexibility is specific to each joint and depends on a number of specific variables, including but not limited to the tightness of specific ligaments and tendons.

fracture: Broken bone. People with osteoporosis, osteogenesis imperfecta, and Paget disease are at greater risk for bone fracture.

frequency: The number of times an exercise or activity is performed. Frequency is generally expressed in sessions, episodes, or bouts per week.

healthy weight: A body mass index (BMI) of 18.5–24.9 is considered a healthy weight, though not all individuals with a BMI in this range may be at a healthy level of body fat; they may have more body fat tissue and less muscle. A person with a BMI of 25–29.9 is considered overweight, and a person with a BMI of 30 or more is considered obese.

heart rate: Reserve is the difference between the resting heart rate and the maximal heart rate.

hydration: The amount of fluid in your body. It is important to replace any fluid your body loses during physical activity.

hypertension: Blood pressure greater than 140 over 90 mmHg (millimeters of mercury). Long-term high blood pressure can damage blood vessels and organs, including the heart, kidneys, eyes, and brain. Also called "high blood pressure."

leisure-time physical activity: A recreational activity generally associated with pleasure and/or health and fitness. Such activities are varied as to type and intensity. Some leisure-time activities are of light intensity such as sitting in a boat fishing; others are of moderate activity, such as low impact aerobics. Those that are classified as vigorous intensity are more strenuous, such as high impact aerobics or running.

metabolism: The chemical changes that take place in a cell or an organism. These changes make energy and the materials cells and organisms need to grow, reproduce, and stay healthy. Metabolism also helps get rid of toxic substances.

moderate-intensity physical activity: On an absolute scale, physical activity that is done at 3.0–5.9 times the intensity of rest. On a scale relative to an individual's personal capacity, moderate-intensity physical activity is usually a 5 or 6 on a scale of 0–10.

muscle-strengthening activity: Physical activity, including exercise that increases skeletal muscle strength, power, endurance, and mass.

nutrition: The taking in and use of food and other nourishing material by the body. Nutrition is a three-part process. First, food or drink is consumed. Second, the body breaks down the food or drink into nutrients.

osteoporosis: Literally means "porous bone." This disease is characterized by too little bone formation, excessive bone loss, or a combination of both, leading to bone fragility and an increased risk of fractures of the hip, spine, and wrist.

overweight: Overweight refers to an excessive amount of body weight that includes muscle, bone, fat, and water. A person who has a body mass index (BMI) of 25–29.9 is considered overweight.

pedometer: A step counter that is worn at the waist or on a person's waistband. It tallies the number of steps a person takes each day. Walking 2,000 steps is equal to about one mile and roughly 100 calories are burned over and above calories for resting metabolism.

physical activity: Any bodily movement that is produced by the contraction of skeletal muscle and that substantially increases energy expenditure.

physical fitness: The ability to carry out daily tasks with vigor and alertness, without undue fatigue, and with ample energy to enjoy leisure-time pursuits and respond to emergencies.

protein: A molecule made up of amino acids. Proteins are needed for the body to function properly. They are the basis of body structures, such as skin and hair, and of other substances such as enzymes, cytokines, and antibodies.

relative intensity: The level of effort required by a person to do an activity. When using relative intensity, people pay attention to how physical activity affects their heart rate and breathing.

steroid: Any of a group of lipids (fats) that have a certain chemical structure. Steroids occur naturally in plants and animals or they may be made in the laboratory.

stimulants: A class of drugs that enhance the activity of monoamines (such as dopamine and norepinephrine) in the brain, increasing arousal, heart rate, blood pressure, and respiration, and decreasing appetite; includes some medications used to treat attention deficit hyperactivity disorder (e.g., methylphenidate and amphetamines), as well as cocaine and methamphetamine.

Glossary of Terms Related to Fitness and Exercise

strength: A health and performance component of physical fitness that is the ability of a muscle or muscle group to exert force.

stretching: Stretching includes movements that lengthen muscles to their maximum extension and move joints to the limits of their extension.

target heart rate: A safe heart rate recommended for fitness workouts; it depends on age and gender. It is the rate you want the heart to work (beats per minute) during a certain activity. You can use it to help determine the intensity of an activity.

vigorous-intensity physical activity: On an absolute scale, physical activity that is done at 6.0 or more times the intensity of rest. On a scale relative to an individual's personal capacity, vigorous-intensity physical activity is usually a 7 or 8 on a scale of 0–10.

vitamin D: A nutrient that the body needs to absorb calcium.

warm-up: A gradual increase in the intensity of exercise to allow physiological processes to prepare for greater energy outputs. Changes include a rise in body temperature, cardiorespiratory changes (i.e., increased heart and ventilation rate), and increase in muscle elasticity and contractility.

weight control: This refers to achieving and maintaining a healthy weight with healthy eating and physical activity.

yoga: An ancient system of practices used to balance the mind and body through exercise, meditation (focusing thoughts), and control of breathing and emotions.

Chapter 51 | Directory of Fitness Resources

GOVERNMENT ORGANIZATIONS

Agency for Healthcare Research and Quality (AHRQ)
5600 Fishers Ln.
7th Fl.
Rockville, MD 20857
Phone: 301-427-1104
Website: www.ahrq.gov

Americans with Disabilities Act (ADA)
950 Pennsylvania Ave., N.W.
Washington, DC 20530-0001
Toll-Free: 800-514-0301
Toll-Free TTY: 833-610-1264
Website: www.ada.gov

Centers for Disease Control and Prevention (CDC)
1600 Clifton Rd., N.E.
Atlanta, GA 30329
Toll-Free: 800-CDC-INFO
(800-232-4636)
Phone: 770-488-1725
Toll-Free TTY: 888-232-6348
Website: www.cdc.gov
Email: hrcs@cdc.gov

Federal Communications Commission (FCC)
45 L St., N.E.
Washington, DC 20554
Toll-Free: 888-CALL-FCC
(888-225-5322)
Phone: 202-418-1122
Toll-Free TTY: 888-TELL-FCC
(888-835-5322)
Toll-Free Fax: 866-418-0232
Website: www.fcc.gov

Federal Occupational Health (FOH)
5600 Fishers Ln., Ste. 600
Bethesda, MD 20814
Toll-Free: 866-4FOH-HLP
(866-436-4457)
Website: www.hhs.gov/about/agencies/asa/foh/index.html

Resources in this chapter were compiled from several sources deemed reliable; all contact information was verified and updated in October 2024.

Federal Trade Commission (FTC)
600 Pennsylvania Ave., N.W.
Washington, DC 20580
Toll-Free: 877-FTC-HELP
(877-382-4357)
Phone: 202-326-2222
Website: www.ftc.gov

National Cancer Institute (NCI)
9609 Medical Center Dr.
Bethesda, MD 20892-9760
Toll-Free: 800-4-CANCER
(800-422-6237)
Website: www.cancer.gov
Email: NCIinfo@nih.gov

National Center for Complementary and Integrative Health (NCCIH)
9000 Rockville Pike
Bethesda, MD 20892
Toll-Free: 888-644-6226
Website: www.nccih.nih.gov
Email: info@nccih.nih.gov

National Heart, Lung, and Blood Institute (NHLBI)
P.O. Box 30105
Bethesda, MD 20824
Toll-Free: 877-NHL-BI4U
(877-645-2448)
Website: www.nhlbi.nih.gov
Email: nhlbiinfo@nhlbi.nih.gov

National Highway Traffic Safety Administration (NHTSA)
1200 New Jersey Ave., S.E.
W. Bldg.
Washington, DC 20590
Toll-Free: 888-327-4236
Phone: 202-366-4000
Toll-Free TTY: 888-275-9171
Website: www.nhtsa.gov
Email: nhtsa.webmaster@dot.gov

National Institute of Arthritis and Musculoskeletal and Skin Diseases (NIAMS)
1 AMS Cir.
Bethesda, MD 20892-3675
Toll-Free: 877-22-NIAMS
(877-226-4267)
Phone: 301-495-4484
Fax: 301-718-6366
Website: www.niams.nih.gov
Email: NIAMSinfo@mail.nih.gov

National Institute of Diabetes and Digestive and Kidney Diseases (NIDDK)
9000 Rockville Pike
Bethesda, MD 20892
Toll-Free: 800-860-8747
Website: www.niddk.nih.gov
Email: healthinfo@niddk.nih.gov

National Institute of Mental Health (NIMH)
6001 Executive Blvd.
MSC 9663
Bethesda, MD 20892-9663
Toll-Free: 866-615-6464
Website: www.nimh.nih.gov
Email: nimhinfo@nih.gov

Directory of Fitness Resources

National Institute on Aging (NIA)
P.O. Box 8057
Gaithersburg, MD 20898
Toll-Free: 800-222-2225
Website: www.nia.nih.gov
Email: niaic@nia.nih.gov

National Institute on Drug Abuse (NIDA)
3 White Flint N., 11601 Landsdown St.
North Bethesda, MD 20852
Phone: 301-443-6441
Website: https://nida.nih.gov

National Institutes of Health (NIH)
9000 Rockville Pike
Bethesda, MD 20892
Phone: 301-496-4000
TTY: 301-402-9612
Website: www.nih.gov

NIH News in Health
9000 Rockville Pike
Bldg. 31, Rm. 5B52
Bethesda, MD 20892
Phone: 301-451-8224
Website: https://newsinhealth.nih.gov
Email: nihnewsinhealth@od.nih.gov

Office of Dietary Supplements (ODS)
6705 Rockledge Dr.
Rm. 730, MSC 7991
Bethesda, MD 20817
Website: https://ods.od.nih.gov
Email: ods@nih.gov

Office of Disease Prevention and Health Promotion (ODPHP)
1101 Wootton Pkwy., Ste. 420
Rockville, MD 20852
Website: https://health.gov/about-odphp/contact-us

Office on Women's Health (OWH)
1101 Wootton Pkwy.
Rockville, MD 20852
Toll-Free: 800-994-9662
Phone: 202-690-7650
Fax: 202-205-2631
Website: www.womenshealth.gov
Email: womenshealth@hhs.gov

U.S. Consumer Product Safety Commission (CPSC)
4330 E.W. Hwy
Bethesda, MD 20814
Toll-Free: 800-638-2772
Toll-Free TTY: 800-638-8270
Fax: 301-504-0124; 301-504-0025
Website: www.cpsc.gov

U.S. Department of Agriculture (USDA)
1400 Independence Ave., S.W.
Washington, DC 20250
Phone: 202-720-2791
Website: www.usda.gov
Email: feedback@oc.usda.gov

U.S. Department of Health and Human Services (HHS)
200 Independence Ave., S.W.
Hubert H. Humphrey Bldg.
Washington, DC 20201
Toll-Free: 877-696-6775
Website: www.hhs.gov

U.S. Department of Veterans Affairs (VA)
810 Vermont Ave., N.W.
Washington, DC 20420
Phone: 202-461-4800
Website: www.va.gov

U.S. Environmental Protection Agency (EPA)
1200 Pennsylvania Ave., N.W.
Washington, DC 20460
Phone: 202-564-4700
Website: www.epa.gov

U.S. Food and Drug Administration (FDA)
10903 New Hampshire Ave.
Silver Spring, MD 20993
Toll-Free: 888-INFO-FDA
(888-463-6332)
Phone: 301-796-8240
Website: www.fda.gov

U.S. National Library of Medicine (NLM)
8600 Rockville Pike
Bethesda, MD 20894
Toll-Free: 888-FIND-NLM
(888-346-3656)
Phone: 301-594-5983
Website: www.nlm.nih.gov
Email: custserv@nlm.nih.gov

PRIVATE ORGANIZATIONS

American Academy of Orthopaedic Surgeons (AAOS)
9400 W. Higgins Rd.
Rosemont, IL 60018-4976
Toll-Free: 800-346-AAOS
(800-346-2267)
Phone: 847-823-7186
Fax: 847-823-8125
Website: www.aaos.org

American College of Sports Medicine (ACSM)
6510 Telecom Dr., Ste. 200
Indianapolis, IN 46278
Phone: 317-637-9200
Fax: 317-634-7817
Website: www.acsm.org
Email: publicinfo@acsm.org

American Council on Exercise (ACE)
9444 Balboa Ave., Ste. 290
San Diego, CA 92123
Toll-Free: 888-825-3636
Phone: 858-576-6500
Fax: 858-576-6564
Website: www.acefitness.org
Email: support@acefitness.org

American Diabetes Association (ADA)
2451 Crystal Dr., Ste. 900
Arlington, VA 22202
Toll-Free: 800-DIABETES
(800-342-2383)
Website: www.diabetes.org
Email: askada@diabetes.org

Directory of Fitness Resources

American Heart Association (AHA)
7272 Greenville Ave.
Dallas, TX 75231
Toll-Free: 800-AHA-USA-1
(800-242-8721)
Website: www.heart.org

American Lung Association (ALA)
55 W. Wacker Dr., Ste. 1150
Chicago, IL 60601
Toll-Free: 800-LUNGUSA
(800-586-4872)
Website: www.lung.org
Email: info@lung.org

American Orthopaedic Society for Sports Medicine (AOSSM)
9400 W. Higgins Rd., Ste. 300
Rosemont, IL 60018
Toll-Free: 877-321-3500
Phone: 847-292-4900
Website: www.sportsmed.org
Email: info@aossm.org

American Physical Therapy Association (APTA)
3030 Potomac Ave., Ste. 100
Alexandria, VA 22305-3085
Toll-Free: 800-999-APTA
(800-999-2782)
Phone: 703-684-APTA
(703-684-2782)
Fax: 703-684-7343
Website: www.apta.org

American Stroke Association (ASA)
7272 Greenville Ave.
Dallas, TX 75231
Toll-Free: 888-4-STROKE
(888-478-7653)
Website: www.stroke.org

Aquatic Exercise Association (AEA)
1618 Ellis St.
Brunswick, GA 31520
Toll-Free: 888-232-9283
Phone: 912-289-3559
Website: https://aeawave.org
Email: info@aeawave.org

Arthritis Foundation (AF)
1355 Peachtree St., N.E., Ste. 600
Atlanta, GA 30309
Toll-Free: 800-283-7800
Phone: 404-872-7100
Website: www.arthritis.org

Athletics and Fitness Association of America (AFAA)
355 E. Germann Rd.
Bldg. 6
Gilbert, AZ 85297
Toll-Free: 800-446-2322
Website: www.afaa.com
Email: customerservice@afaa.com

Bone Health and Osteoporosis Foundation (BHOF)
251 18th St., S., Ste. 630
Arlington, VA 22202
Toll-Free: 800-231-4222
Website: www.bonehealthandosteoporosis.org
Email: info@bonehealthandosteoporosis.org

Cleveland Clinic
9500 Euclid Ave.
Cleveland, OH 44195
Toll-Free: 800-223-2273
Phone: 216-444-2200
Website: https://my.clevelandclinic.org

HealthyWomen (HW)
P.O. Box 336
Middletown, NJ 07748
Toll-Free: 877-986-9472
Phone: 732-530-3425
Website: www.healthywomen.org
Email: info@healthywomen.org

IDEA Health & Fitness Association
9921 Carmel Mountain Rd., #126
San Diego, CA 92129
Toll-Free: 800-999-IDEA
(800-999-4332)
Phone: 858-535-8979
Website: www.ideafit.com
Email: contact@ideafit.com

International Fitness Association (IFA)
12472 Lake Underhill Rd., Ste. 341
Orlando, FL 32828
Phone: 407-579-8610
Website: www.ifafitness.com

Move United
451 Hungerford Dr., Ste. 608
Rockville, MD 20850
Phone: 301-217-0960
Website: https://moveunitedsport.org

National Alliance for Youth Sports (NAYS)
5670 Corporate Way
West Palm Beach, FL 33407
Toll-Free: 800-688-KIDS
(800-688-5437)
Fax: 561-684-2546
Website: www.nays.org

National Center on Health, Physical Activity and Disability (NCHPAD)
3810 Ridgeway Dr.
Birmingham, AL 35209
Toll-Free: 866-866-8896
Website: www.nchpad.org
Email: nchpad@uab.edu

National Recreation and Park Association (NRPA)
22377 Belmont Ridge Rd.
Ashburn, VA 20148-4501
Toll-Free: 800-626-NRPA
(800-626-6772)
Website: www.nrpa.org
Email: customerservice@nrpa.org

National Strength and Conditioning Association (NSCA)
1885 Bob Johnson Dr.
Colorado Springs, CO 80906
Toll-Free: 800-815-6826
Phone: 719-632-6722
Fax: 719-632-6367
Website: www.nsca.com

Directory of Fitness Resources

Society of Health and Physical Educators (SHAPE) America
P.O. Box 225
Annapolis Junction, MD 20701
Toll-Free: 800-213-7193
Phone: 703-476-3400
Fax: 703-476-9527
Website: www.shapeamerica.org

Women's Sports Foundation
247 W. 30th St., 5th Fl.
New York, NY 10001
Toll-Free: 800-227-3988
Website: www.womenssportsfoundation.org
Email: info@WomensSportsFoundation.org

INDEX

INDEX

INDEX

Page numbers followed by "n" refer to citation information; by "t" indicate tables; and by "f" indicate figures.

A

absolute intensity, defined 91
active lifestyle
   emotional development 63
   family fitness 175
   healthy aging 222
   physical activity 58, 110
   walking 203
activity levels
   physical activity 52
   pregnancy 97
   walking 203
   weight management 34
aerobic activity
   cancer 342
   chronic disease 108
   coronary heart disease 94
   described 3, 90, 103
   flexibility exercises 227
   osteoarthritis 293
   overview 187–190
   overweight and obesity 308
   physical activity 25, 57, 75, 129
   staying active 173
   weight management 34
aerobic exercise
   cravings 350
   endurance exercise 13

   healthy aging 108
   physical activity 78
   strength training 222
Agency for Healthcare Research and Quality (AHRQ), contact information 383
alcohol
   adult care 330
   bicycle safety 121
   healthy meal 140
   hydration and health 262
   meditation and mindfulness 242
   physical activity 52
   physical health 21
   sleep habits 356
   wellness care 372
American Academy of Orthopaedic Surgeons (AAOS), contact information 386
American College of Sports Medicine (ACSM), contact information 386
American Council on Exercise (ACE), contact information 386
American Diabetes Association (ADA), contact information 386
American Heart Association (AHA), contact information 387
American Lung Association (ALA), contact information 387
American Orthopaedic Society for Sports Medicine (AOSSM), contact information 387

American Physical Therapy Association (APTA), contact information 387
American Stroke Association (ASA), contact information 387
Americans with Disabilities Act (ADA), contact information 383
anabolic steroids
    asthma 333
    bodybuilding 274
    overview 269–273
anemia, healthy weight 36
anxiety
    brain health 19
    cancer 343
    inactive lifestyle 346
    managing weight 101
    meditation and mindfulness 242
    mental health 254
    mind and body practices 231
    obesity 167
    physical activity 10, 23, 89, 115
    physical exercise 5
    social support 329
    swimming 197
    tabulated 20t
    weight management 33
    youth health 79
Aquatic Exercise Association (AEA), contact information 387
arm exercises, physical activity 133
arthritis
    cardiac rehabilitation 316
    obesity 167
    overview 321–324
    physical activity 9, 114, 130
    physical exercise 5
    physical inactivity 44
    walking 204
    water-based exercise 197
    weight management 33
Arthritis Foundation (AF), contact information 387

assistive devices, physical activity 118
asthma
    childhood obesity 166
    overview 331–334
    xanthines 270
Athletics and Fitness Association of America (AFAA), contact information 387

B

balance activities
    bone-strengthening activity 4
    physical activity 323
balance training
    managing chronic conditions 112
    muscle-strengthening activity 108
    physical activity 342
    resistance training exercises 325
balanced eating
    active lifestyle 263
    managing weight 104
bicycle safety
    crashes 213
    exercising outdoors 120
bicycling
    aerobic activity 92, 188
    cardiovascular activity 250
    endurance activity 14
    overview 211–212
    physical activity 58, 310
    physical exercise 6
    weight management 35t
blood pressure
    exercise 115
    exercising outdoors 290
    food myths 41
    goal setting 149
    heart disease risk 94
    hypertension 295
    lifelong health 75
    managing diabetes 335
    mind and body practices 231

Index

blood pressure, *continued*
   physical activity 9, 60, 102
   physical health 20
   strength exercises 221
   sympathomimetics 270
   weight management 33
BMI *see* body mass index
body composition
   physical activity 75
   resistance training 219
body mass index (BMI)
   defined 307
   healthy weight 36
   managing weight 101
   overview 164–167
   physical inactivity 43
body weight
   body mass index (BMI) 164
   energy balance 170
   muscle-strengthening activity 79, 93, 103
   osteoarthritis 293
   physical activity 11, 60
   resistance training exercises 325
   strength exercises 6, 15
   strength training 220
bodybuilding
   overview 274–276
   weight loss products 184
bodyweight exercises
   physical activity 157
   strength training 222
bone health
   cancer 343
   osteoporosis 324
   physical activity 11, 60
   resistance training 219
   swimming 197
Bone Health and Osteoporosis Foundation (BHOF), contact information 387
bone-strengthening activity, described 4

brain health
   Alzheimer disease (AD) 28
   lifelong health 75
   physical activity 19
   weight management 33
breastfeeding, hydration and health 261
brisk walking
   aerobic activity 90, 187
   arthritis 322
   cardiovascular activity 250
   hippocampal atrophy 27
   managing chronic conditions 112
   muscle-strengthening activity 78
   physical activity 12, 300
   staying active 139
   walking 203
   weight management 34
   weight-bearing exercises 325
building strength, physical exercise 5

C

calorie intake
   exercise 115
   healthy weight 37
   heart health 163
   physical activity 12
   weight management 33
calorie requirements, tabulated 169t
calories
   active lifestyle 263
   bicycling 212
   cardiovascular activity 250
   food myths 40
   healthy lifestyle 83
   healthy meal 140
   heart health 163
   physical activity 312, 337
   physical fitness 69
   tabulated 35t
   vigorous activity 36
   wearable technology 361
   weight management 33

cancer
　aerobic activity 90, 187
　endurance exercise 13
　exercise 115
　hypertension 295
　inactive lifestyle 346
　mind and body practices 231
　mood regulation 22
　obesity 167
　overview 339–344
　physical activity 9, 33, 79, 255
carbohydrate
　food myths 40
　healthy eating plan 69
　physical activity 337
cardiac rehabilitation, overview 315–317
cardiorespiratory fitness
　aerobic activity 91
　lifelong health 75
　physical activity 11, 79
　pregnancy 98
cardiovascular activity, described 249
cardiovascular fitness, physical therapy 328
Centers for Disease Control and Prevention (CDC)
　contact information 383
　publications
　　adding physical activity as an adult 131n
　　BMI FAQs 167n
　　cardiac rehabilitation 317n
　　child activity 58n
　　getting started with physical activity 157n
　　health benefits of physical activity for children 60n
　　healthy eating tips for a healthy weight 142n
　　high school parents 287n
　　lowering risk for women 94n
　　overcoming barriers to physical activity 157n
　　overweight and obesity and health 102n
　　physical activity 81n
　　physical activity and arthritis 324n
　　physical activity and weight and health 35n
　　physical activity for child 59n
　　physical inactivity older adults 45n
　　positive parenting for preschoolers 62n
　　pregnant and postpartum activity 99n
　　prompts to encourage physical activity 152n, 154n
　　school health guidelines 68n
　　water and healthier drinks 262n
cholesterol
　coronary heart disease 94
　health monitoring 368
　heart health 163
　inactive lifestyle 346
　managing diabetes 335
　managing weight 101
　obesity 167
　physical activity 173
　physical health 20
　physical inactivity 80
　type 2 diabetes 294
chronic disease
　body mass index (BMI) 166
　cancer 342
　family fitness 175
　healthy eating 264
　lifelong health 75
　managing chronic conditions 107
　mind and body practices 231
　osteoarthritis 293
　physical activity 11, 51, 89, 155, 300
　physical inactivity 43

Index

chronic pain, mind and body
  practices 231
Cleveland Clinic, contact
  information 388
cognition, tabulated 19t
cognitive function
  brain health 19
  cancer 343
  emotional benefits 10
  hippocampal atrophy 26
  physical activity 53, 75, 111
  physical exercise 5
cognitive health, brain
  health 20
competitive sports, vigorous-
  intensity activity 35
concussion, overview 285–287
cool down
  aerobic activity 188
  exercise 14
  social support 156
  workout 253
coronary heart disease
  aerobic activity 95
  moderate-intensity aerobic
    activity 90
  overweight
    individuals 101
  physical activity 94
  physical inactivity 45t
coronavirus 2019 (COVID-19)
  digital health care 373
  obesity 167
  outdoor activities 362
  physical activity 24
COVID-19 see coronavirus 2019
cycling
  cravings 350
  exercise habits 146
  exercising outdoors 120
  physical activity 323
  strength training 222

D

dehydration
  health monitoring 368
  hydration and health 261
  physical activity 337
  yoga 236
depression
  aerobic activity 90
  anabolic steroid 273
  brain health 19
  cardiac rehabilitation 316
  healthy living 299
  inactive lifestyle 346
  mental health 23, 254
  mind and body practices 231
  obesity 166
  physical activity 11, 60
  physical exercise 5
  sleep deficiency 354
  social support 329
  swimming 197
  tabulated 20t
  weight management 33
  youth health 79
diabetes
  endurance exercise 13
  healthy weight 36
  heart health 163
  managing chronic conditions 112
  mental health 82
  overview 335–338
  physical activity 130, 254, 310
  physical health 20
  physical inactivity 45
  water-based exercise 197
diet
  caffeinated drinks 262
  cardiac rehabilitation 315
  chronic disease prevention 67
  coronary heart disease 94
  exercise 111
  food myths 40

diet, *continued*
    lifestyle modifications 328
    physical activity 24
    physical health 21
    physical inactivity 80
    strength training 223
    walking 250
    weight loss myths 181
    weight management 34
dietary supplements
    overview 266–269
    resistance training 219
    steroids 274
    sympathomimetics 270
disease prevention
    heart disease 161
    physical activity 52, 67
Division of Occupational Health and Safety (DOHS)
    publication
        2023 top fitness trends 362n
duration
    brain health 20t
    defined 250
    exercise-induced asthma 332
    exercising outdoors 289
    mood regulation 23
    physical activity 12, 75, 116
    pregnancy 96
    social support 156

E

early death
    anabolic steroid 272
    managing weight 101
    physical activity 155
    social support 329
    walking 203
employee wellness programs, physical activity services 68
endurance activities *see* aerobic exercise

energy
    aerobic activity 91
    cardiac rehabilitation 316
    comfort foods 142
    cravings 351
    exercise and well-being 111
    healthy foods 69
    healthy weight 36, 83
    hiking 206
    menstrual cycle 99
    mood regulation 23
    physical activity 3, 9
    physical exercise 5
    staying active 132
    strength training 222
    sugary drinks 262
    sympathomimetics 270
    weight management 33
energy balance, overview 168–170
energy levels
    cravings 351
    healthy weight 36
    menstrual cycle 99
    mental health 254
    mood regulation 23
    physical activity 111, 132
    physical exercise 5
exercise
    asthma medications 333
    fitness trainers 180
    flexibility activity 4
    healthy sleep habits 356
    hippocampal atrophy 26
    keeping bones healthy 325
    menstrual cycle 99
    muscle-strengthening activity 173
    overview 111–114
    physical activity 21, 77
    quitting smoking 349
    sports injuries 279
    strength training 222
    stretching 16

Index

exercise, *continued*
  vigorous activity 35
  workout 256
  yoga 10
exercise equipment
  group fitness instructors 179
  physical activity 347
  weight loss products 182
  workout mistakes 253
exercise routines, bone health 326
exposure
  cancer risk 342
  exercising outdoors 289
  healthy life 299
  swimming 199
  wellness tourism 365

F

fat
  anabolic steroids 270
  comfort foods 142
  food myths 40
  healthy diet 21
  healthy foods 264
  heart disease 161
  inactive lifestyle 345
  ketoacidosis 337
  lifelong health 75
  managing weight 37
  obesity 167
  physical activity 60
  resistance training 219
Federal Communications
  Commission (FCC), contact
  information 383
Federal Occupational Health (FOH),
  contact information 383
Federal Trade Commission (FTC)
  contact information 384
  publication
    weight loss ads 184n

fitness apps
  physical activity plan 312
  routine chores 72
fitness classes, indoor activities 176
fitness goals
  physical activity plan 312
  physical activity roadblocks 135
fitness trainers 179
fitness zone, physical
  appearance 153
flexibility
  aerobic activity 188
  anabolic steroids 271
  cooling down 251
  exercise 13
  overview 225–228
  physical activity 3, 51
  resistance training 336
  sports injuries 279
  stretching 16
flexibility activities
  defined 4
  physical activity 3
flexibility training
  aerobic activity 187
  physical fitness 225
fracture
  bicycling safety 213
  mindfulness 223
  osteogenesis imperfecta (OI) 327
  osteoporosis 324
  sports injuries 280
frequency
  bone-strengthening
    activities 75
  cardiovascular activity 250
  exercise-induced asthma 332
  mind and body practices 231
  physical activity 12, 116
  qigong 238
functional training, physical
  activity 145

G

girlshealth.gov
   publication
      importance of physical activity 83n
goal setting 147
gymnastics
   age-appropriate activities 58
   physical activity goals 59

H

HBP *see* high blood pressure
health
   active lifestyle 110
   aerobic activity 91
   Alzheimer disease (AD) 27
   chronic disease prevention 67
   diabetes 336
   energy drinks 262
   exercise 346
   exercising outdoors 289
   food myths 40
   healthy eating habits 266
   healthy foods 139
   healthy weight 36
   managing weight 101
   mood regulation 22
   overweight individuals 167
   physical activity 3, 52, 89, 309
   physical fitness 225
   strength exercises 7
   swimming 197
   target heart rate zone 161
   wellness care 371
   workout mistakes 252
   yoga 236
health benefits
   exercise 10
   goal setting 147
   healthy aging 107
   mental health 25
   physical activity 52, 75
   sleep deprivation 355
   sports injuries 285
   swimming 199
   weight management 33
health education, healthy eating 66
health monitoring, smart devices 367
health promotion, tai chi 237
healthy diet
   cardiac rehabilitation 316
   daily steps 250
   physical health 21
   schools 66
healthy eating
   parents and caregivers 266
   postpartum 98
   school guidelines 65
   yoga 235
healthy fats, gaining weight 37
healthy foods
   active lifestyle 263
   people with disabilities 299
   schools 66
   staying active 139
   teenagers 69
healthy lifestyle
   coronavirus 2019 (COVID-19) 362
   older adults 111
   osteogenesis imperfecta (OI) 328
   people with disabilities 299
   screen time 83
healthy living
   cardiac rehabilitation 315
   diabetes 335
   people with disabilities 299
healthy weight
   aging 36
   body mass index (BMI) 164, 307t
   coronary heart disease 94
   eating right 139
   older adults 111
   physical activity 9, 34, 254

Index

healthy weight, *continued*
   postpartum 98
   screen time 83
   teenagers 69
   walking 203
HealthyWomen (HW), contact
   information 388
heart disease
   aerobic activities 187
   aging 36
   body mass index (BMI) 164
   endurance exercise 13
   healthy eating 264
   hypertension 295
   inactive lifestyle 346
   older adults 111
   osteoarthritis 293
   overweight individuals 101
   physical activity 9, 33, 79, 114
   physical inactivity 161
   tai chi 231
   type 2 diabetes 294
   walking 203
   water-based exercise 197
   women 93
   see also coronary heart disease
heart health 163
high blood pressure (HBP)
   childhood obesity 166
   cognitive health 20
   coronary heart disease 95
   heart health 163
   inactive lifestyle 346
   overweight individuals
      101, 310
   sleep 356
   type 2 diabetes 294
   walking 204
high-intensity interval training (HIIT),
   tabulated 79t
HIIT *see* high-intensity interval
   training

hiking
   aerobic activity 103
   calories 35t
   moderate-intensity aerobic 78t
   older adults 109
   overview 205–207
   overweight individuals 311
   vigorous activity 6
   vigorous-intensity aerobic 78t, 92t
hippocampal atrophy 26
home gyms 25
hormone
   bodybuilding products 274
   menstrual cycle 99
   sleep 355
hydration
   athletic performance 269
   overview 261–263
   physical activity 337

I

IDEA Health & Fitness Association,
   contact information 388
immune system
   asthma 332
   cancer 342
   inactive lifestyle 345
   swimming-related illnesses 199
inactive lifestyle, overview 345–347
inactivity, tabulated 44t
indoor cycling 138
insulin resistance, physical inactivity 80
International Fitness Association
   (IFA), contact information 388
interval training *see* high-intensity
   interval training

J

jogging
   aerobic activity 70, 103, 187
   calories 36t

Fitness and Exercise Sourcebook, Seventh Edition

jogging, *continued*
   endurance exercise 13
   healthy bones 325
   moderate activity 6
   older adults 109
   shared enjoyment 137
   urban areas 120
   vigorous-intensity activity 34, 92t

L

lifestyle modification, osteogenesis imperfecta (OI) 328
lung capacity, quitting smoking 350

M

martial arts
   flexibility exercises 227
   overview 191–193
   physical activity 78
meditation
   complementary health practices 232
   mind and body practices 231
   overview 241–243
   tai chi 10
   wellness tourism 363
MedlinePlus
   publications
      health risks of an inactive lifestyle 347n
      physical exercise 6n
menopause
   breast cancer 340
   yoga 234
mental disorders, physical activity 101
mental health
   brain health 31
   cardiac rehabilitation 315
   chronic disease prevention 67
   exercise 10

   healthy eating 72
   mood regulation 23
   obesity 166
   osteoarthritis 293
   physical activity 25, 111, 129
   pregnancy 237
   sleep deprivation 353
   water-based exercise 197
   wellness tourism 364
metabolism
   cancer risk 342
   dietary supplements 268
   inactive lifestyle 345
   physical health 22
   resistance training 219
   strength training 223
mindful eating, wellness tourism 365
mindfulness
   overview 241–243
   staying strong 223
moderate-intensity physical activity
   aerobic activity 336
   bone health 326
   cardiovascular exercise 95
   depicted 130f
   described 34
   managing chronic conditions 108
   physical activity myths 41
   physical activity plan 312
   pregnancy 98
   vigorous physical activity 12
   wayfinding 152
mood disorders, mood regulation 23
Move United, contact information 388
muscle soreness
   cooling down 249
   physical activity 310
muscle-strengthening activity
   defined 4
   depicted 130f
   described 92

Index

muscle-strengthening activity, *continued*
   multicomponent physical activity 110
   physical activity 145
   pregnancy 97

N

National Alliance for Youth Sports (NAYS), contact information 388
National Cancer Institute (NCI)
   contact information 384
   publication
      physical activity and cancer 344n
National Center for Complementary and Integrative Health (NCCIH)
   contact information 384
   publications
      meditation and mindfulness 243n
      mind and body practices 232n
      mind and body practices for children and teens 233n
      qigong 240n
      tai chi 238n
      yoga 236n
National Center on Health, Physical Activity and Disability (NCHPAD), contact information 388
National Heart, Lung, and Blood Institute (NHLBI)
   contact information 384
   publications
      asthma and physical activity in school 334n
      balance food and activity 170n
      being active for a healthy heart 190n
      everyday ideas to move more 138n
      guidelines for healthy and safe swimming 199n
      making physical activity a habit 147n
      making physical activity routine 187n
      martial arts 193n
      physical activity 4n
      physical activity and your heart 163n, 189n
      physical activity recommendations 61n
      preventing swimming-related illnesses 200n
      reducing screen time 86n
      sleep deprivation and deficiency 357n
      swimming and health 198n
      walking for better health 204n
National Highway Traffic Safety Administration (NHTSA)
   contact information 384
   publication
      bicycle safety 216n
National Institute of Arthritis and Musculoskeletal and Skin Diseases (NIAMS)
   contact information 384
   publications
      exercise for bone health 327n
      sports injuries 281n
National Institute of Biomedical Imaging and Bioengineering (NIBIB)
   publication
      smartwatch data and clinical test prediction 369n
National Institute of Diabetes and Digestive and Kidney Diseases (NIDDK)
   contact information 384

National Institute of Diabetes and
   Digestive and Kidney Diseases
   (NIDDK), *continued*
   publications
      health tips for adults 104n
      healthy living with
         diabetes 338n
      staying active at any size 313n
      tips to help you get active 136n
National Institute of Mental Health
   (NIMH), contact information 384
National Institute on Aging (NIA)
   contact information 385
   publications
      cognitive health and older
         adults 22n
      exercise and physical activity
         benefits 10n
      exercise for healthy aging 149n
      exercises for health and physical
         ability 16n, 188n
      exercising with chronic
         conditions 28n
      fitness for life 115n
      maintaining a healthy weight 37n
      physical activity and Alzheimer-
         related hippocampal
         atrophy 27n
      safety tips for exercising
         outdoors for older
         adults 121n
      strength training and
         aging 224n
National Institute on Drug Abuse
   (NIDA), contact information 385
National Institutes of
   Health (NIH)
   contact information 385
   publications
      benefits of walking 205n
      hydrating for health 263n
      light exercise and memory 31n
      light physical activity and heart
         disease risk in older women
         123n
      maintaining muscle 221n
      osteogenesis imperfecta (OI)
         330n
      physical activity and depression
         symptoms 23n
      steps 133n
National Recreation and Park
   Association (NRPA), contact
   information 388
National Strength and Conditioning
   Association (NSCA), contact
   information 388
NIH News in Health, contact
   information 385
nutrition
   balanced diet 269
   cardiac rehabilitation 315
   fitness trainers 180
   healthy eating 67
   physical activity 25
nutritious foods, active lifestyle 263
nutritious school meals, school meal
   program 66

O

obesity
   body mass index (BMI) 164
   coronary heart disease 94
   exercise habits 145
   food myths 41
   inactive lifestyle 346
   lifelong health 75
   lifestyle modifications 328
   managing weight 102
   overweight 307
   physical activity 60, 79
   social health 67
   strength training 223

Index

obesity, *continued*
    wellness tourism 363
    yoga 234
obstacle courses, outdoor activities 177
Office of Dietary Supplements (ODS)
    contact information 385
    publication
        dietary supplements for exercise and athletic performance 269n
Office of Disease Prevention and Health Promotion (ODPHP)
    contact information 385
    publications
        eating healthy 266n
        getting active 174n
        new exercise habit 147n
        Physical Activity Guidelines for Americans, Second Edition 12n, 19n, 54n, 60n, 78n, 93n, 98n, 148n, 296n
        physical activity implementation strategies for older adults 119n
        promoting family fitness 178n
Office on Women's Health (OWH)
    contact information 385
    publication
        physical activity and menstrual cycle 101n
OI *see* osteogenesis imperfecta
osteoarthritis
    chronic conditions 293
    managing chronic conditions 107
    mind and body practices 231
    obesity 167
    physical activity 101
    physical fitness 225
    tai chi 237
osteogenesis imperfecta (OI), overview 327–330
osteopenia, bone health 325

osteoporosis
    bone health 324
    exercise 114
    inactive lifestyle 346
    lifelong health 75
    physical activity 9
    physical inactivity 80
    weight management 33
outdoor activities
    body weight training 361
    described 362
    exercise 138
    family fitness 176
    physical activity 114
overcoming obstacles, tabulated 157t
overload, muscle-strengthening activity 93

P

parks and recreation, staying active 112
pedometer
    physical activity plan 312
    sports 177
    walking 250
physical activity
    aerobic activity 187
    asthma 331
    cancer 339
    cooling down 249
    disease prevention 52
    goal setting 147
    healthy life 300
    healthy sleep habits 356
    heart disease 93
    hippocampal atrophy 26
    menstrual cycle 99
    mental health 82
    muscle-strengthening 78
    osteoarthritis 293
    overview 3–7

physical activity, *continued*
   physical education 62
   social support 156
   sports injuries 279
   staying active 117
   weight management 33, 168
physical education
   academic success 80
   overview 62–64
   physical activity services 68
physical fitness
   bone-strengthening 78
   dietary supplements 269
   exercise-induced asthma 332
   flexibility 225
   managing chronic conditions 107
   physical activity 25
   physical education 62
   quitting smoking 349
   resistance training 219
physical function
   cancer 343
   disease prevention 53
   healthy aging 107
   managing weight 101
   osteoarthritis 293
   physical activity 12
physical health
   cognitive health 20
   cooling down 251
   exercise 10
   physical activity 24, 116
   sleep deprivation 353
physical therapist
   cardiac rehabilitation 315
   muscle-strengthening activity 303
   physical activity 324
   sports injuries 282
physical therapy
   managing arthritis 322
   physical activity 329
   sports injury 281

Pilates
   defined 189
   flexibility exercises 227
playground equipment
   child safety 61
   muscle-strengthening 79
pregnancy
   overview 96–99
   qigong 240
   tai chi 237
   water intake 261
   yoga 235
premature mortality, *Physical Activity Guidelines for Americans* 51
professional development, health and fitness 68
protein
   being physically active 21
   eat healthier 140
   food myths 40
   foods and beverages 69
   strength training 223
   supplements 267
public spaces, barriers to physical activity 116

Q

qigong
   health and wellness 233
   overview 238–240
QOL *see* quality of life
quality of life (QOL)
   adults and older adults 11
   arthritis 322
   being physically active 89, 133
   brain health 19
   cancer 295
   disease prevention 53
   managing chronic conditions 107, 293
   managing weight 101

Index

quality of life (QOL), *continued*
   mind and body practices 231
   obesity 166
   tabulated 20t
   tai chi and qigong 237

R

recovery
   concussion 286
   danger signs 287
   healthy weight 36
   heart health 315
   nutrition and exercise 271
   physical activity 96
   strength training basics 220
   wellness tourism 365
recreational activities
   being physically active 58, 147
   fitness trainers 180
   flexibility 226, 251
   health benefits 197
rehabilitation
   defined 284
   osteogenesis imperfecta (OI) 327
   overview 315–317
   sports injury 281
   tai chi 237
relative intensity, aerobic activity 92
resilience, youth mental health 25
resistance bands
   joint-friendly physical activity 323
   muscle-strengthening activity 93, 103
   strength exercises 6, 14, 79t
   strength training 222, 250, 362
resistance training *see* strength training
rest periods, wellness tourism 365
risk factors
   arthritis 321
   children and adolescents 75

coronary heart disease 94
endometrial cancer 340
hypertension 295
sports injury 279
swimming 198
type 2 diabetes 294

S

saturated fat
   defined 264
   foods and beverages 69
   heart health 163
   Nutrition Facts label 265
self-esteem
   childhood obesity 166
   exercise-induced asthma 332
   osteogenesis imperfecta (OI) 329
   physical activity 5, 25, 82, 254
self-monitoring 361
skiing, tabulated 78t
skipping
   aerobic and bone-strengthening activity 77
   preschoolers 60
   tabulated 79t
sleep, tabulated 20t
sleep deprivation
   described 353
   healthy sleep habits 357
sleeping habits 72
Smokefree Women
   publication
      moving 96n
Smokefree.gov
   publications
      cravings and exercise 351n
      smoking and workout 350n
Society of Health and Physical Educators (SHAPE) America, contact information 389

sodium
	foods and beverages 69
	nutrients and ingredients 264
sports injury, overview 279–287
sports medicine 267
squats
	arthritis 321
	flexibility exercises 227
	muscle-strengthening activity 109
	resistance training 220
	strength exercises 6
stamina, osteogenesis imperfecta
	(OI) 329
steroids
	bodybuilding products 275
	fraudulent and adulterated
		products 269
	see also anabolic steroids
strength training
	aerobic activity 188
	diabetes 336
	exercise 14
	fitness trends 361
	joint-friendly physical activity 323
	muscle-strengthening activity 103
	overview 219–224
	overweight individuals 311
stress management, yoga 235
stretching exercises 226
stroke
	being active 310
	bodybuilding products 274
	exercise 5, 9, 114
	healthy weight 36
	inactive lifestyle 346
	moderate-intensity aerobic
		activity 90
	older adults 45t
	older women 122
	overweight individuals 101, 167
	physical activity 11, 33, 203
	physical health 356

substance abuse 299
swimming
	aerobic activity 90, 103, 187, 336
	cardiovascular activity 250
	children 58
	cravings 350
	endurance exercise 13
	family fitness 177
	joint-friendly physical activity 323
	moderate-intensity aerobic 78t
	older adults 109
	osteoarthritis 294
	osteogenesis imperfecta (OI) 329
	overcoming obstacles 158t
	overview 197–200
	people with disabilities 302
	physical activity 3
	shared enjoyment 138
	vigorous physical activity 36t
	vigorous-intensity aerobic 78t, 92t

T

tai chi
	balance exercises 15, 325
	brain health 29
	emotional and cognitive benefits 111
	emotional benefits 10
	flexibility exercises 227
	joint-friendly physical activity 323
	martial arts 192
	mind and body practices 231
	muscle-strengthening activity 109
	older adults 223
	osteoarthritis 294
	overview 237–238
target heart rate
	depicted 162f
	described 161
team sports
	family fitness 176
	mental health 25
	older adults 114

Index

telehealth, coronavirus 2019 (COVID-19) 373
treatment options
    arthritis 322
    sleep deprivation 357
tumbling, preschoolers 60

U

U.S. Bureau of Labor Statistics (BLS)
    publication
        fitness trainers and instructors 180n
U.S. Consumer Product Safety Commission (CPSC), contact information 385
U.S. Department of Agriculture (USDA), contact information 385
U.S. Department of Health and Human Services (HHS), contact information 385
U.S. Department of Veterans Affairs (VA), contact information 386
    publication
        pumping up physical activity 227n, 251n
U.S. Environmental Protection Agency (EPA)
    contact information 386
    publication
        exercise and air pollution 290n
U.S. Food and Drug Administration (FDA)
    contact information 386
    publication
        bodybuilding products and risks 276n
U.S. Forest Service (USFS)
    publication
        hiking 207n

U.S. Government Publishing Office (GPO)
    publication
        performance triad 220n
U.S. National Library of Medicine (NLM), contact information 386

V

vigorous-intensity physical activity
    cardiovascular exercise 95
    depicted 130f
    heart rate 34
    school-aged youth 75
vitamin D 141, 265

W

walking
    aerobic activity 57, 90, 103, 187, 336
    Alzheimer disease (AD) 26
    arthritis 322
    balance activity 4
    bone-strengthening activity 4
    cold weather 121
    craving 350
    daily steps 250
    emotional benefits 10
    endurance exercise 13
    energy balance 168
    health benefits 308
    independent physical activity 177
    menstrual cramps 100
    moderate-intensity activity 92t
    moderate-intensity aerobic 78t
    moderate-intensity physical activity 34
    older adults 109, 115
    osteoporosis 325
    overcoming obstacles 157t
    overview 203–205

walking, *continued*
   postpartum period 98
   rural areas 120
   social support 146
   urban areas 120
warm-up, described 249
wearable devices
   fitness goals 312
   wellness care 371
wearable technology, described 361
weight control, meditation or
   mindfulness 242
weight lifting
   moderate physical activity 35t
   self-efficacy 146
   young people 80
weight loss
   ephedra 270
   muscle-strengthening activity 93
   myths and scams 181
   older adults 223
   physical activity 33
   postpartum period 98
   walking 203
   wearable technology 361
weight management
   energy balance 168
   osteogenesis imperfecta (OI) 328
   physical activity 33
   sugar alternatives 262
wellness programs 68

wellness tourism, overview 363–366
Women's Sports Foundation, contact
   information 389
workouts
   accountability 146
   brain health 29
   cooldown 251
   daily routine 147
   dementia 28
   menstrual cycle 100
   self-efficacy 145
   social support 146

Y

yoga
   aerobic activity 109
   brain health 29
   complementary health 232
   emotional and cognitive
      benefits 111
   flexibility activity 4, 227
   group fitness 179
   health benefits 189
   mind and body practices 231
   mindfulness 223
   muscle strengthening 79t
   overview 233–236
   resistance training 220
   self-efficacy 146
   wellness tourism 363